I0426661

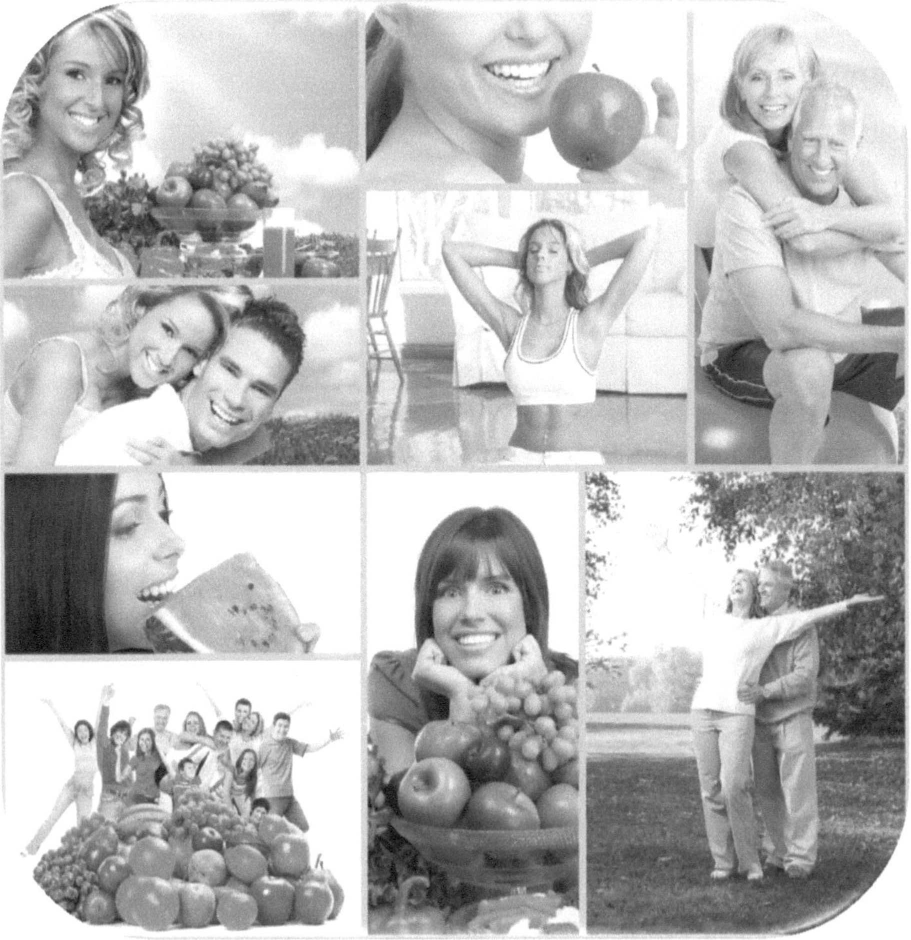

Contents

INTRODUCTION

In the twenty-first century and living in the land of plenty, as you probably are if you're reading this book, you have many and varied temptations leading you away from good feeding habits. You are constantly bombarded by the food industry wanting to make a profit with never a thought for your health or physique. They want your money. Your body is your responsibility.

However, congratulations are in order. By starting to read this book, you have taken an important step towards achieving a leaner, healthier body. You are about to read a cut-the-crap version of how to eat for maximising your fitness and having optimum energy levels. If you are serious about enhancing your physique and being healthier and fitter all at the same time, you need to know how to feed your body to progress beyond your wildest dreams.

The Fitness Wizards have a combined total of seventy years of personal experience and progressing exercisers; we know that what, how much, and when you feed have a big effect on performance and recovery. Get it right and adopt some good habits, and you will have plenty of energy to train and recover from each session ready for the next. Get it wrong, and you will be in for a world of pain and will simply not be able to keep up the pace. The term overtraining could just as easily be called "under-feeding" or "inappropriate feeding". Your state of mind, training, feeding, and resting are the big four for progression in any sport or physique-enhancing endeavour. Whether it is a weight training Programme or any other sport, the rules for feeding are similar. The Great Body Bible weight training programme is featured in the bestselling book The Great Body Bible by the Fitness Wizards, available in paperback and e-book form from the major stockists. Google it to find the most cost effective 700+ page training tool you will ever buy.

We are always amazed by how many exercisers sabotage their progress by leaving feeding and diet to chance. Most follow the more-is-better philosophy, and because of this, many athletes are just plain fatter than they deserve after all of their hard work in the gym. Knowing what to take on board before, during, and after working out will allow you to get

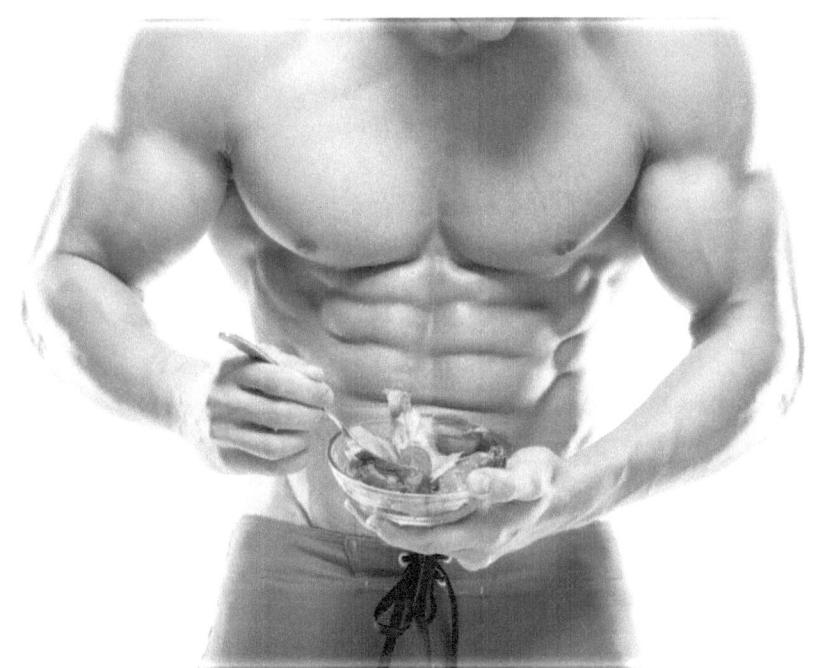

the most out of your training programmes. Whether you weight train in the gym, run, cycle, swim, or do any other sport or active pastime, you will benefit from making some easy changes to your feeding habits. These will result in improved performance, and you will look and feel better.

Judging by the number of times I get asked the question "How do I lose fat and gain muscle?" This is the most desired result. These goals can be achieved by the correct state of mind, careful feeding, consistent training, and good rest. Assuming responsibility for your feeding is the first step. Nobody is going to do it for you – unless you have a personal trainer on call all day. But for all of the rest of us, self-reliance is the key. Julie and I are fortunate that we both have the same or similar fitness and physique goals, but not having your significant others on board can make life difficult. Fail to plan your feeds properly and you will never get lean, no matter how hard you train. In this book you will learn how to adapt your eating and training to get the physique you want.

I am constantly asked whether there are special or magic foods or supplements that can enhance your performance or make you burn more body fat. I will mention a few of these sports foods and drinks and let you know which are worth the money and which are not. But I will say now there is nothing that will compensate for poor state of mind, feeding, training, or resting, and any useful aid will only help when those four habits are firmly in place.

I will tell you how to tailor your feeds to your weight training programme. This information will also be transferable and can be adapted for those of you that do other sports. Introducing active body feeding will make a startling difference to your physique. I would say that changing feeding habits leads to more happy customers than any training programme ever could on its own. Progress comes to those that can conquer their dietary needs and lose any attachments to junk foods.

The mind leads training, feeding, plenty of good sleep, and stress-free relaxation. The perfect combination for optimum peace of mind, physique, health, and fitness. With those habits in place, it will all happen perfectly.

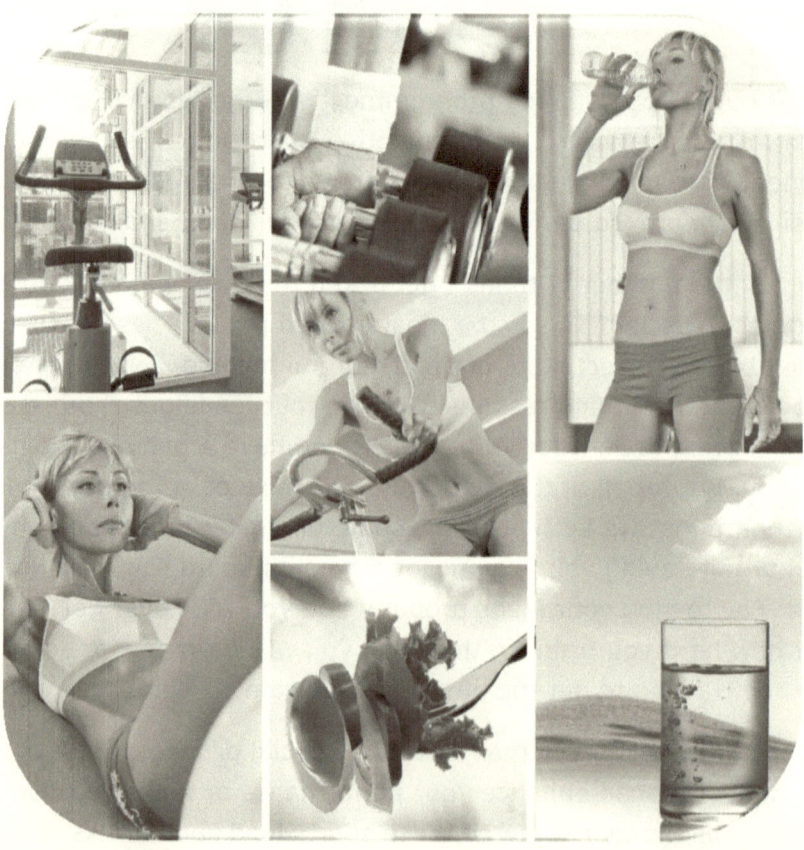

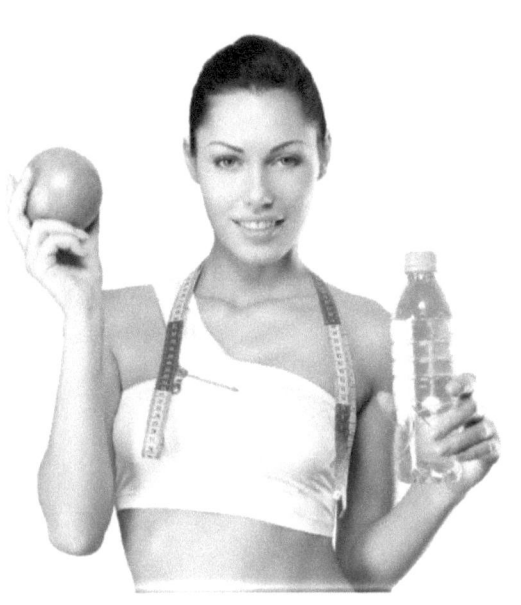

WHAT TO FEED ON

If you are looking to develop your fitness and physique using a weight training programme, you will need five-star fuel. Your needs will be vastly different from [those of] the average couch potato. Everyone needs to balance their feeds to avoid illness, but as an athlete – and that is what you have become if you are actively training on a regular basis – you will need feeds that meet the tough demands of your training programme, plus your life away from the gym and any specific goals you may have, such as muscle gain or fat loss. Get the balance right and you will have energy and feel more vital for your training and for your life. Just to add, as I will throughout this book – adequate sleep and stress management are also vital. Correct feeding will help with both.

FOODS FOR FITNESS

It is important that you get more vitamins, minerals, antioxidants, and phytonutrients than non-active people – nutrients that are vital for keeping your body in peak health. I will list the food groups and portions that will be the foundation for your feeding plan, to help you construct a healthier diet that is better suited to an active lifestyle. As you will be feeding as often as six times per day, you can gauge how many feeds will include that particular food group each day. There is also a difference for muscle gain and fat loss, depending on your primary goal at that time. The ratios remain the same but increase for muscle-gain programmes. It is easier to view this as the portions being larger for a muscle-gain programme, maybe even twice the size, and a ratio of two to one.

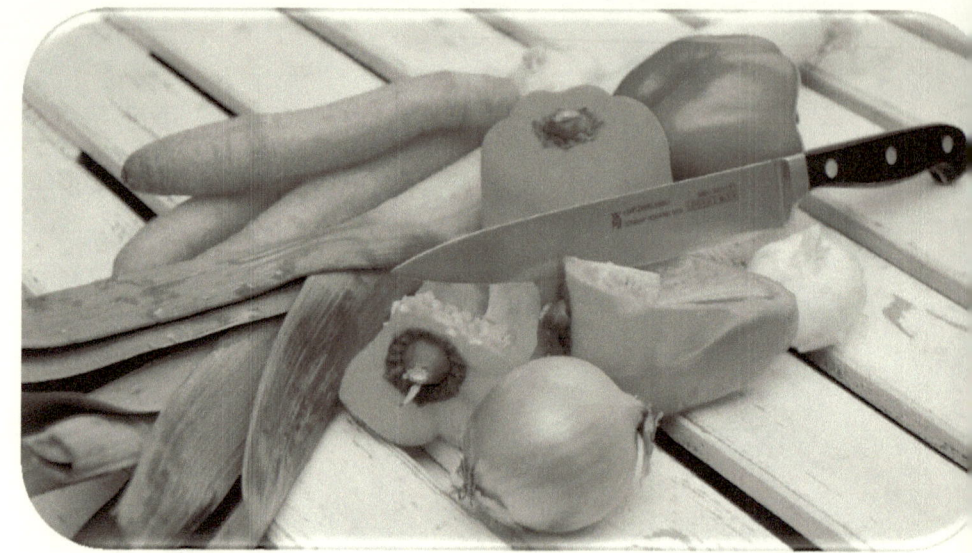

• Fruit: 2–4 portions • Vegetables: 3–5 portions • Carbohydrate-rich foods: 4–6 portions • Protein-rich foods: 6+ portions • Calcium-rich foods: 2–4 portions • Healthy Fats: 2 portions • Junk food: 0–1 portion

It is important that the balance is maintained, as there are important nutrients in each food group that will optimise your health. The one exception to this rule is for a pre-contest bodybuilder, when the required look dictates that certain extreme dietary practices are followed. In this case, periods of zero or at least very low carbs and food group cycling are recommended. However, one can achieve an extremely high level of physique by just following normal feeding as described above. I myself have won a local show after following a healthy, balanced plan. Other extreme plans do take an extreme amount of dedication, and one never feels great. At times the difference in physique can be marginal. In my case, it has been worse at times, when I have followed what can only be described as a wacky feeding plan.

The more varied your feed the more likely you are to get the nutrients you need. It may seem easier to stick to the same feeds day after day, but you could end up missing some vital nutrients. Eating lots of one or two kinds of food, whatever it may be, doesn't make a balanced diet. In fact, let's use bodybuilding as an example. Large amounts of protein are considered as essential in bodybuilding circles. Remembering that protein sales are what that particular sport depends on, I have on occasion run out of protein and not been able to replenish my stocks. I have noted at these times that I have become leaner and harder without losing any strength. This resulted solely from not supplementing protein via shakes but rather just having it in each feed. That points to fat loss and muscle retention, a tightening of my physique caused by consuming less protein. Bodybuilders beware! You are likely to get fat on too much protein, just as you would on any other macro nutrient – and it will cost you much more for the privilege! Keep that balance, and don't believe all the hype from people sponsored by the protein manufacturers or those who stand to profit from your overconsumption of protein products.

PORTION SIZES

What constitutes a portion size? It is not an exact science, but the following list will allow you to estimate your feed sizes. We are generally either eating to be healthy while gaining and maintaining good muscle size, or we are stripping for a show. One of the tricks we use is having different-sized plates for each period. If we want to lose fat, we use smaller plates; it does stop one overfeeding whilst not having to worry about portion sizes. I like to make my life as easy as possible. All portion sizes and amounts are for natural athletes, but they should be adjusted upwards should this not be the case. However, all ratios should remain the same. Fad diets and feeding schedules are not necessary and can be detrimental to one's health.

• Fruit: A piece about the size of a tennis ball. Usually one medium fruit, two small fruits, or a handful of berry-type fruit

• Vegetables: The amount you can hold in one hand

• Carbohydrate-rich foods: A handful of rice or cereals, a fist-sized baked potato, or two slices of bread

• Calcium-rich food: a cup of milk (skimmed), a carton of yogurt, or a tiny amount of cheese.

• Protein-rich foods: Meat/poultry/fish the size of a deck of cards, two eggs, or a protein shake as per tub

• Healthy fats: two teaspoons olive oil or similar, two tablespoons nuts and seeds, or a piece of oily fish

ABOUT FRUITS AND VEGETABLES

Fruit: 2–4 portions per day; Vegetables: 3–5 portions per day

Fruits and vegetables provide vitamins, minerals, fibre, and phytonutrients, which are vital for peak health. Decent levels boost immunity and protect from disease. Fruits and vegetables are best when grown locally in season, not imported, and (stating the obvious) not damaged at all. Fruits and vegetables are at their best when bought and used fresh. Nutritional content deteriorates in time with exposure to light and air. Overcooking can have the same results.

• Buy seasonal varieties, when they are cheaper and fresher. • Washing fruits and vegetables is wise – just to be sure.

• The best way to avoid chemical residue is to buy organic.

• Frozen can be a good option, as the freezing process ensures a high level of nutrition. What that level is depends on how fresh they are when frozen. I tend to have some faith and believe that they are very fresh

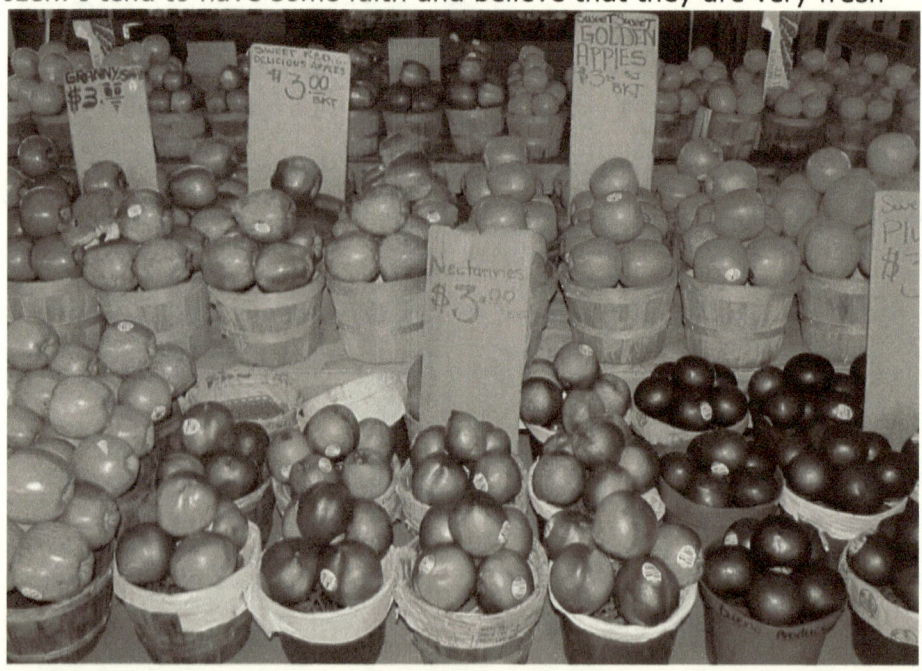

when frozen to preserve the appearance for future sales. Belief is half the battle, the placebo effect.

ABOUT PHYTONUTRIENTS

Phytochemicals are compounds that occur naturally in plants. They are powerful antioxidants that work with vitamins and minerals to protect the body from disease and degeneration; they boost immunity, fight harmful bacteria, and ward off viruses. Eating your portions of fruit and vegetables will ensure you are amply supplied.

The general term for anything in your body that causes damage is free radicals, and simply put, antioxidants destroy free radicals. Some foods are more effective at this. Fruit and vegetables have been tested for their ability to combat harmful free radicals. ORAC stands for Oxygen Radical Absorbance Capacity. These are the preferable options for your health. Prunes and raisins appear higher because they contain no water.

TOP SCORING ANTI-OXIDANT FRUIT AND VEGETABLES	
Fruit / Veg	ORAC - score
Prunes	5,770
Raisins	2,830
Blueberries	2,400
Blackberries	2,036
Kale	1,770
Strawberries	1,540
Spinach	1,260
Raspberries	1,220
Brussels Sprouts	980
Plums	949
Broccoli	890
Beets	840
Oranges	750
Red Grapes	739
Red peppers	710
Cherries	670
Kiwi fruit	602
Pink Grapefruit	483
Onions	450
Corn	400
Aubergines	390

Mixing the colours of your fruit and veg will ensure you get a wide range of phytonutrients and great health protection.

• Green: watercress, broccoli, cabbage, rocket, Brussels sprouts, leafy salad, curly kale

• Red/Purple: plums, aubergines, cherries, beetroot, red grapes, strawberries, blackberries, blueberries, tomatoes

• Yellow/Orange: peaches, apricots, nectarines, oranges, yellow peppers, squash • White/Yellow: onions, garlic, apples, pears, celery

• Brown/Green: beans, lentils, bean sprouts, nuts, seeds, tea

ABOUT VITAMINS AND MINERALS

Vitamins support the immune system, help the brain function, and are vital to the conversion of food to energy. They are needed for healthy skin and hair and controlling hormones and growth. Water-soluble vitamins, such as B and C, can't be stored and are needed every day from your feeds.

Minerals are needed for structure and regulation, including bone strength and regrowth. Your bones are regenerating constantly. Haemoglobin manufacture, fluid balance, and muscle contraction all depend on minerals. If the food forms your building blocks, the vitamins and minerals are the cement that keeps it all together and happening perfectly.

ABOUT CARBOHYDRATES

Carbs: 4–6 portions per day

Carbs include bread, breakfast cereal, rice, pasta, porridge oats, beans, lentils, and potatoes. Carbohydrates are the preferred fuel source of our bodies for exercise and for everyday living. Once in your body, carbs are

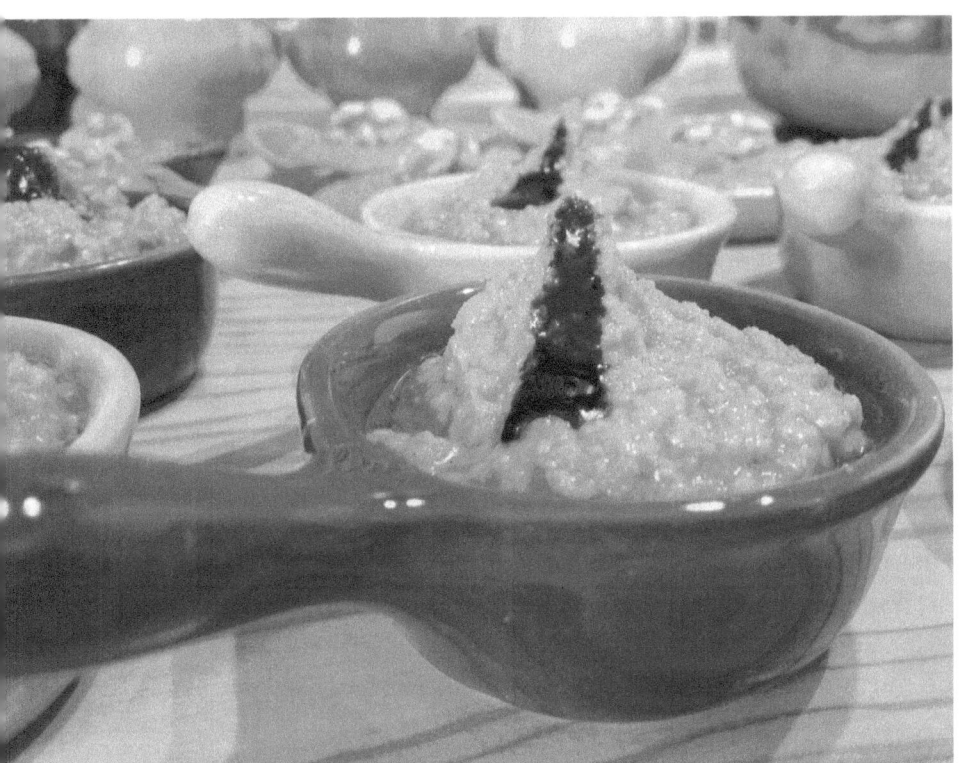

:ored as glycogen. If you work out regularly, you have to keep your
lycogen levels high to enable you to train hard. Low glycogen levels
esult in low energy and poor performance. Complex carbs also offer
bre, B vitamins, and minerals, such as iron. Use whole wheat and
nrefined carbs – wholemeal bread, breakfast cereals, pasta, and rice –
ather than the white versions, which have much of the nutritional
ontent stripped away. Variety is again the way to go, as most people
ist go for wheat products and often develop a wheat allergy. Use oats,
rown rice, and starchy vegetables such as sweet potatoes and regular
otatoes. Porridge oats is a great way to start the day, and I often use it
ade with skimmed milk or a made up protein shake as a feed later in
e day also. Once you have tried chocolate protein porridge you will love

.

ll carbs are turned into glucose eventually, but some are fast and some
re slow and some are in between. All carbs are not equal. Some foods
roduce a rapid swing in blood-sugar levels, while other foods have a
ore gradual effect. This is measured by something called the glycaemic

index (GI). Foods are ranked from 1–100, with glucose having a GI of 100. This index tells you how foods will affect your blood-sugar levels.

Foods that break down quickly during digestion have the highest GIs. Foods that break down more slowly, releasing glucose into the bloodstream gradually, are said to have a lower GI. Fast carbs are generally refined starchy foods – potatoes, corn flakes, white bread, and white rice – along with sugary foods such as soft drinks, cakes, biscuits, and sweets. Slower carbs are generally less refined – beans, lentils, porridge, coarse-grain bread, muesli, and fruit and dairy products. It is quite logical that the more fibrous foods will take longer to digest, thus releasing glucose into the bloodstream slower. Consult the GI table for an idea of which are the slow and the fast carbs.

Fast carbs give only a short-lived energy boost; that is then followed by a drop in energy levels. It is not hard to see why this is not ideal for exercise and how a more constant and gradual release of energy would be much more advantageous for training and recovery.

The Glycaemic Index and Carb Content Of Food			
Food	Size	Carbs(g)	GI
Breakfast Cereals			
Muesli	50g	34	56
Weetabix	40g	30	69
Shredded wheat	45g	31	67
Rice crispies	30g	27	82
Cornflakes	30g	26	84
Cheerios	30g	23	74
Porridge(water)	160g	14	42
Grains and Pasta			
Brown rice	180g	58	76
White rice	180g	56	87
Spaghetti	220g cooked	49	41
Basmati rice	60g	48	58
Macaroni pasta	230g cooked	43	45
Instant noodles	230g cooked	30	46
Bread			
Pizza	115g	38	60
White bread	36g	18	70
Wholemeal bread	38g	16	69
Crackers/Crispbreads			

Rice cakes	8g	6	85
Biscuits and Cakes			
Sponge Cake	60g	39	46
Muffin	68g	34	44
Digestive	15g	10	59
Shortbread	13g	8	64
Oatmeal	13g	8	55
Rich Tea	10g	8	55
Vegetables			
Chips	165g	59	75
Old boiled potatoes	175g	30	56
Mashed potatoes	180g	28	70
Sweet potatoes	130g	27	54
New boiled potatoes	175g	27	62
Jacket potatoes	180g	22	85
Sweetcorn	85g	17	55
Parsnip	65g	8	97
Peas	70g	7	48
Carrots	60g	3	49
Pulses			
Baked beans	205g	31	48
Lentils	160g	28	26
Chickpeas	140g	24	33
Red kidney beans	120g	20	27
Fruit			
Banana	100g	23	55
Raisins	30g	21	64
Pear	160g	16	38
Apricot dried	40g	15	31
Grapes	100g	15	46
Apple	100g	12	38
Orange	208g	12	44
Mango	75g	11	55
Cherries	100g	10	22
Pineapple	80g	8	66
Peach	121g	8	42
Kiwi fruit	68g	6	52
Plum	55g	5	39
Apricot	40g	3	57
Drinks			
Fanta	375ml	51	68
Lucozade	250ml	40	95
Isostar	250ml	18	70

Squash diluted	250ml glass (50ml concentrate)	14	66
Snacks			
Tortillas/corn chips	50g	30	72
Crisps	30g	16	54
Peanut	50g	4	14
Dairy products			
Low fat fruit yoghurt	150g	27	33
Skimmed milk	300ml	15	32
Whole milk	300ml	14	27
Ice cream	60g	14	61
Confectionary			
Mars bar	65g	43	68
Milk chocolate	54g	31	49
Muesli bar	33g	20	61
Drinks			
Apple juice	160ml	16	40
Orange juice	160ml	14	46
Sugars			
Honey	17g	13	58
Glucose	5g	5	100
sucrose	5g	5	65

There is no need to cut out high-glycaemic foods altogether. The key is to eat them with protein or healthy fat to lower the overall glycaemic effect, to slow down the digestion. Eating like this gives a more consistent and steady energy supply, less fat storage, and better appetite control. For example, eat a bowl of cereal (high GI) with skimmed milk (low GI). This slows down digestion and gives you a slower burn, exactly what you need.

ABOUT CALCIUM-RICH FOODS

Calcium: 2–4 portions per day

Think calcium; think dairy products, like milk, cheese, and yogurt. Lower-fat options would be best. Cheese is something that we love, but we tend to leave it out of any serious feeding plan. Calcium is needed for strong bones and teeth, plus protein and B vitamins. If you want to avoid dairy, you can choose almonds, dark-green veg, tinned fish with bones included, and calcium-fortified products like pulses and figs.

Protein: 6+ portions per day

Intense and regular trainers need more protein than inactive people. This is vital when you train with weights or any other strength and power activities. Without enough protein, you will not recover or will take longer to recover, and your progress will be slower or non-existent. Include protein rich food with every feed: lean meat, poultry, fish, eggs, soya, Quorn, and protein shakes for convenience immediately after exercise, with some added carb powder to speed recovery. Again, the added benefits are B vitamins, zinc, and iron. Vegetarians may include lentils and dairy against their protein sources. There are many protein supplements on the market, as discussed before. Used sparingly they can be convenient and can aid recovery when eating a solid meal is not practical.

If you work out three or more times per week, you will need between 1.2 and 1.8 g of protein per kg of body weight daily. This may not be as much as the protein vendors tell you, but it's still worthy of consideration. A 70-kg natural athlete will need 84–126 g of protein daily. That works out at

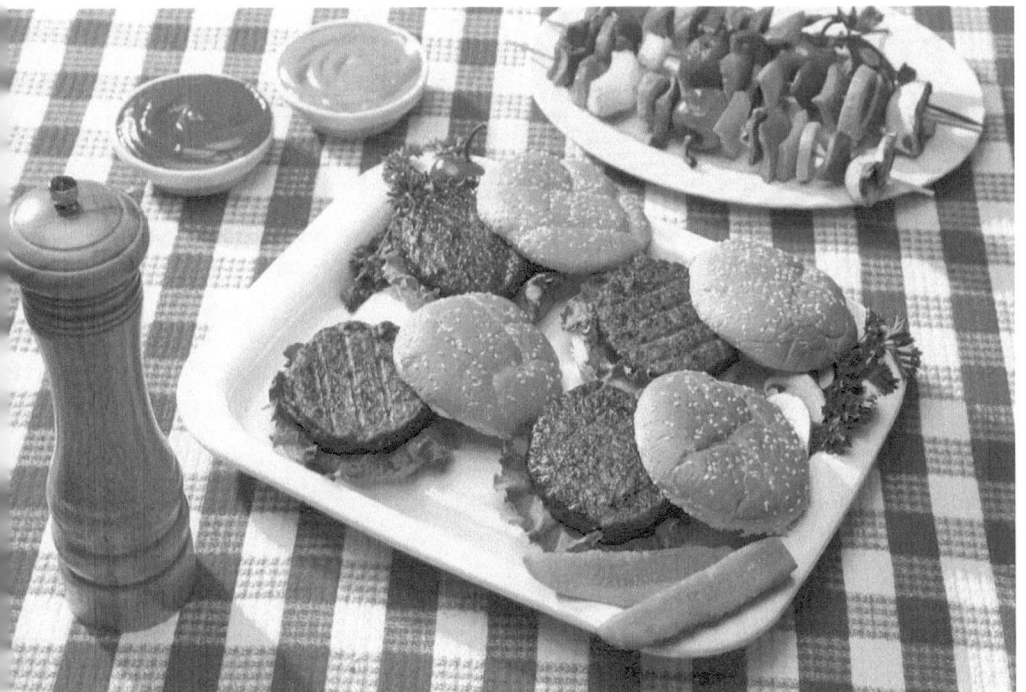

about 25 per cent of your calorie intake; remember that too much may make you fat. Not enough protein can cause fatigue and slow recovery after workouts. Without enough protein, you won't be able to build a lean, strong body. We find that if you are trying to gain muscle, say go from 70–75 kg, then you need to eat as if you are already 75 kg, and so on.

ABOUT HEALTHY FATS

Healthy fats: 1–2 portions per day

EFA: Essential fatty acids, called omega-3 and omega-6, can improve endurance as well as protect against heart disease. Found in nuts, rapeseed oil, olive oil, flaxseed oil, sunflower oil, and oily fish, they are essential for regular exercisers. A good-quality protein supplement may actually contain EFAs as a little added bonus. The following may help:

• A portion of oily fish twice a week: mackerel or salmon

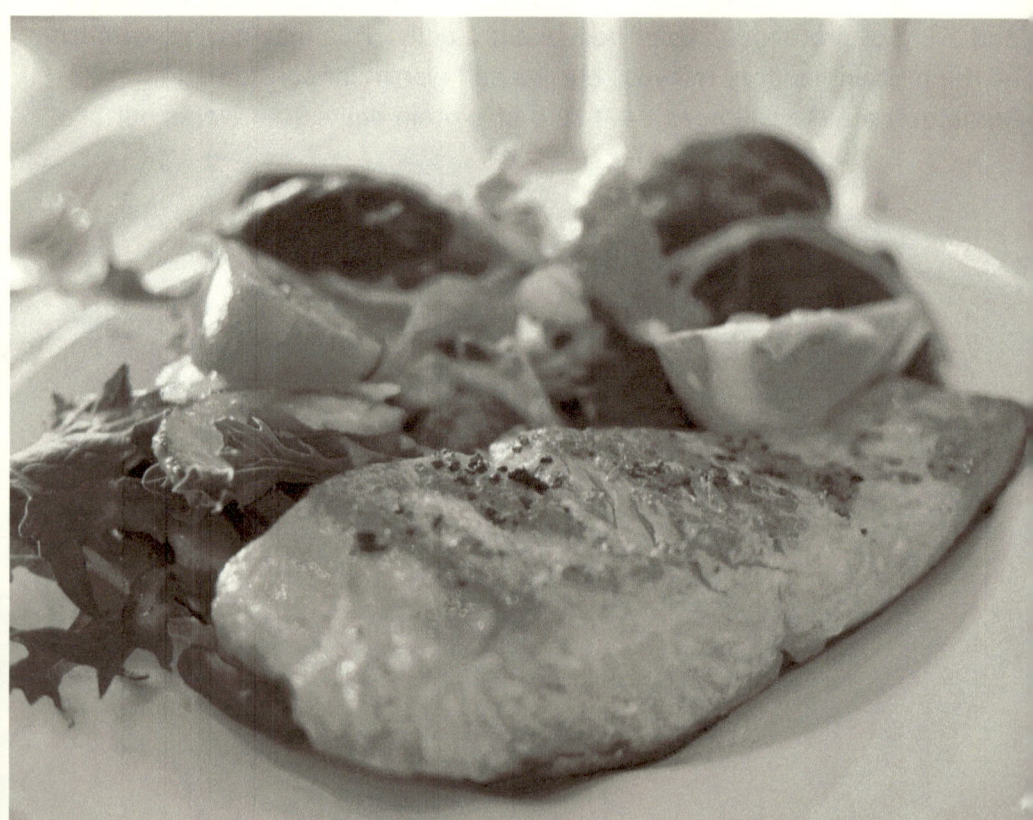

A heaped tablespoon of nuts or seeds per day

A tablespoon of one of the following oils daily: rapeseed, extra virgin olive, flax seed, walnut, sesame, or a blend

A fish oil supplement

Nut butters. These will also contain these oils but beware of the calorie contents. They are rather high.

Healthy fats lower blood cholesterol levels and thus lower the risk of heart disease. A lack of either omega will result in dry and scaly skin. These fats are particularly beneficial for regular exercisers, because they can help you get leaner. Research shows that omega 3 increases the delivery of oxygen to exercising muscles, optimising your aerobic capacity, increasing your endurance, and ultimately, helping burn more fat. They also speed recovery after hard training and reduce inflammation and joint stiffness.

ABOUT JUNK FOODS

We recommend as little as possible each day. Your results may depend on this very discipline.

Junk foods contain not much nutrition but loads of calories. They are addictive, and the producers know it. You are their junk-food-eating puppet as long as you let them offload this crap and control your life. They contain artery-clogging saturated fat and hydrogenated fats. Avoid them as far as possible. The odd indulgence won't kill you, but moderation is the key. If you are in control of your body and feeding, then you can indulge occasionally. If not, then it is better that you steer clear and lose your taste for them altogether.

ABOUT WATER

Get into the habit of drinking water all day long. Have frequent drink breaks, and aim for at least eight glasses a day – and more when it is hot or when you exercise. It is better to drink little and often rather than to drink all in one go, as it encourages urination and greater loss of fluid.

FEEDING BEFORE TRAINING

To be honest, active feeding is about having nutrients on board 24/7 as you are either recovering or about to train. A good feeding plan isn't something you do in bits and pieces; it is optimum nutrition all of the time. There are, however, a few points you need to know about what and when to eat in relation to your workout. This can make a big difference to your energy, your performance, and the amount of fat you burn.

What you eat the day before and during the several hours before your workout dictates how much energy you will have during the workout and how well you will perform. If, for instance, you work out every other day, you will always be recovering from the last or preparing for the next workout, so you can see good feeding is paramount all of the time. The carbs in your food are converted to glycogen and stored in your muscles. This can be compared to filling your car up with fuel before a long journey. You need to ensure you have enough fuel in your tank (muscles before you set off (work out). The amount of carbs an intense trainer will need is around 4–7 g of carbs for every kg of body weight. Seriously intense training athletes may need as much as 10 g/kg. The table below tells you approximately how much carbohydrate you need according to your activity level. An example would be, if you weigh 65 kg and work out three to five hours a week, you should aim for 260–325 g of carbs each day. The glycaemic index table gives you an idea of how many carbs are in certain foods.

How much carbohydrate?	
Activity level	**Grams of carbs/kg/day**
3-5 hrs./week	**4-5**
5-7 hrs./week	**5-6**
1-2 hrs./day	**6-7**
2-4 hrs./day	**7-8**
More than 4 hrs./day	**8-10**

A good way to tell if you are consuming enough carbs is by noting how energetic you feel during your workouts. Too little carbs makes you feel fatigued and lethargic, with a pervading empty feeling during exercise. To use the car analogy again, it's a bit like a car that is very low on fuel, chugging along just before stopping completely. Increasing your carbs by 50–100 g per day should boost your energy enough without making you fat. Listen to your body and get in harmony with how you feel, as it can tell you lot if you just look to the signs. Overeating will not increase your energy levels any further. Instead, you may actually feel heavy, full, and strangely enough, more lethargic. The two feelings may be close; make sure you diagnose the right problem. It is a matter of listening to your own body and getting the balance right between too little and too much carbohydrate.

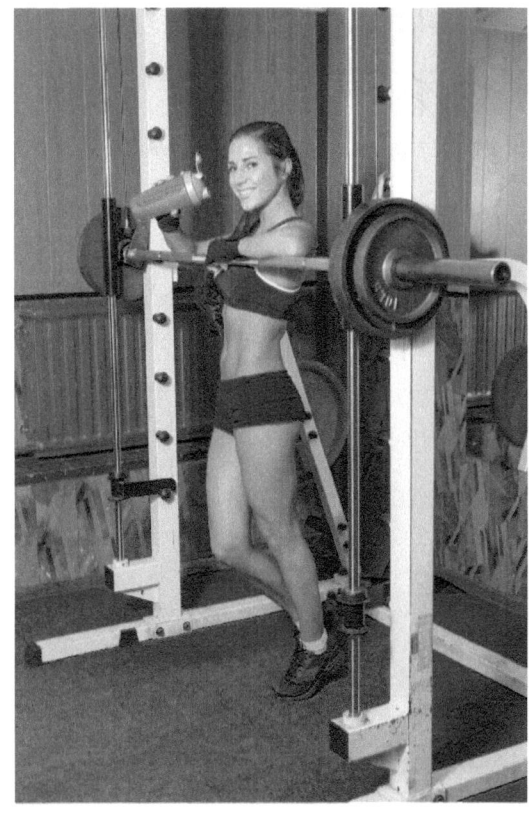

What you eat immediately before training will not affect your muscle glycogen levels. Rather, it will increase your blood-sugar levels, giving you more energy for training and possibly increasing your endurance.

In an ideal world, you should aim to have a meal between two and four hours before a workout. That way you have digested enough not to feel full or hungry yet still have enough fuel for an intense session.

Researchers have discovered that eating a high-carb, low-fat meal three hours before you exercise allows you to exercise longer and perform better. However, this study was comparing three hours with six hours before, so there is no surprise there. My own personal experience has shown me that I need to eat within two hours of training. If I train first thing in the morning, I consume porridge made with skimmed milk about an hour before, and I find that is fine for me. Remember to listen to what the experts say, and then find what works for you based on that knowledge. There are definite behaviours to avoid. Don't eat a big meal right before you work out, and don't train on empty, either. It's a myth that starving before exercise makes you burn more fat. You need five-star fuel for a five-star workout and the physique to match. The following are good reasons to develop good feeding habits before your intense training:

• Train empty and you may become light-headed, weak, and shaky. These are signs of low blood-sugar levels and will certainly stop you from training. When your brain does not get enough fuel, you'll feel faint, lose concentration, and risk injury.

• A full glycogen store with steady blood sugar levels will allow you to train longer and harder. Emptiness equals early fatigue.

• You burn fat when you can train with more intensity and for a longer time. No carbs doesn't mean you will burn fat, as your body burns muscle/protein when there are no sugars available. You will end up losing hard-earned muscle instead of fat.

• The only way you will keep up with the pace in a competitive environment is to fuel correctly. Train empty and you will be the one lagging behind, struggling to keep up with the pace.

• You need to actually get to the gym. When you haven't eaten, or you've eaten too much, you feel lethargic and unmotivated. In that state, and many of you know what I mean, it is hard to get psyched to do anything, and the excuses start flowing thick and fast. Eating a healthy snack at the right time will reduce the temptation to skip your workout.

If you do work out in the morning, it all depends on how much time you have between rising and training. I have found through experience that I can have porridge and skimmed milk an hour before and have a great workout. I do not always feel like the porridge at 5 a.m., but once I start to eat there is not a problem. Many experts would say that is too close to training, but I have no problems at all. I also drink tea. Alternatively, if you wake up a couple of hours beforehand, you will have time to have a light breakfast or snack, such as some cereal, toast, fruit, yogurt, energy bar or, indeed, a bowl of porridge. Drink at least 300 ml of water or even diluted juice before your morning workout. This will help to rehydrate you after many hours with no drinks (while you were sleeping).

Eating too soon before a workout could give you a stitch. If that happens after you have tried a few different breakfast options, even a small meal replacement shake will reduce the risk of dehydration during your workout. If you can't eat anything at all, make sure that you eat plenty the day before and for your breakfast after your workout. I did this for many years; I would have just a cup of tea and then work out, and whilst it is not ideal, I was fine and made good progress. I would not choose to do it now. The science weighs heavily on eating before training, and I can manage perfectly eating one hour before. See what works best for you.

BEST FOODS BEFORE A WORKOUT

Slow-burning, or low-glycaemic, foods that produce a gradual rise in blood sugar are the best bet in your pre-training feed. This will keep you going for longer, with a nice stream of sustained glycogen, and will help avoid problems of low blood sugar during long training sessions.

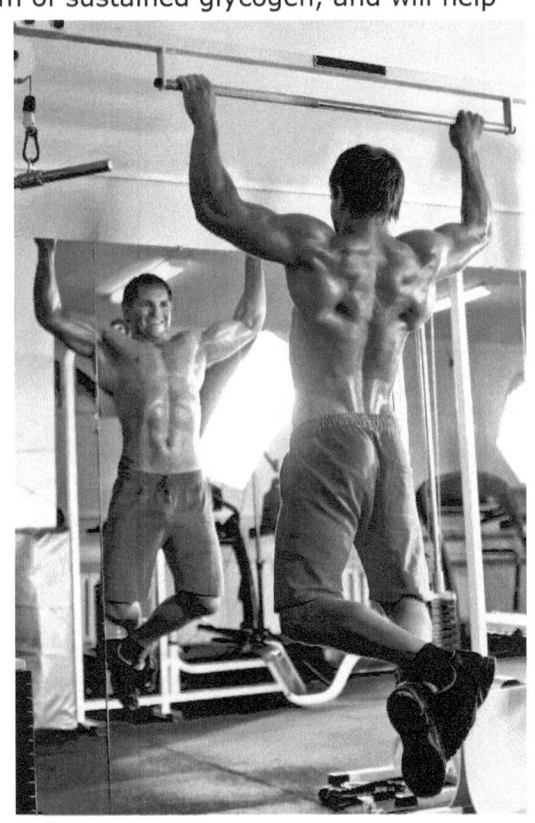

Either eat foods with a low glycaemic index score or combine your carbs with protein or fat, or protein and fat. I give some suggestions below.

PRE-WORKOUT MEALS

Two to four hours before exercise

• Sandwich/roll/bagel/wrap filled with chicken, fish, cheese, egg, or peanut butter

• Jacket potato with beans, cheese, tuna, coleslaw, or chicken

- Pasta with tomato-based sauce and cheese

- Macaroni with cheese and salad chicken, or fish with rice and veg

- Porridge with skimmed milk

- Wholegrain cereal with milk or yogurt

- Fish pie

- Beef chilli and rice

- Stir-fry prawns with noodles

PRE-WORKOUT SNACKS

One to two hours before

- Fresh fruit

- Dried apricots or sultanas

- Smoothie • Yogurt

- Meal replacement shake

- Energy bar

- Cereal/breakfast bar

- Fruit loaf

- Banana cake

- Diluted fruit juice

STAYING HYDRATED

A few tips on hydration

• Dark urine is a sure sign you are low on fluid. Drink until your urine is light yellow coloured. Note also that certain strong supplemental vitamins can cause very dark urine. You can watch your money going down the toilet. Buy weaker vitamins or ensure your food has you covered with a full spectrum of vitamins, minerals, and trace elements.

Drink before you become thirsty. Thirst comes at a time when you will have already lost 2 per cent of your body weight as water. If you relied on thirst as your indicator to drink, you would only ever be 50–75 per cent hydrated.

Drink at least two glasses of water, or about 400–600 ml, two to three hours before your workout. This is the amount recommended by scientists.

Carry a bottle everywhere you go – if you have room with your phone permanently attached to your body. It is a good habit to develop. Drink

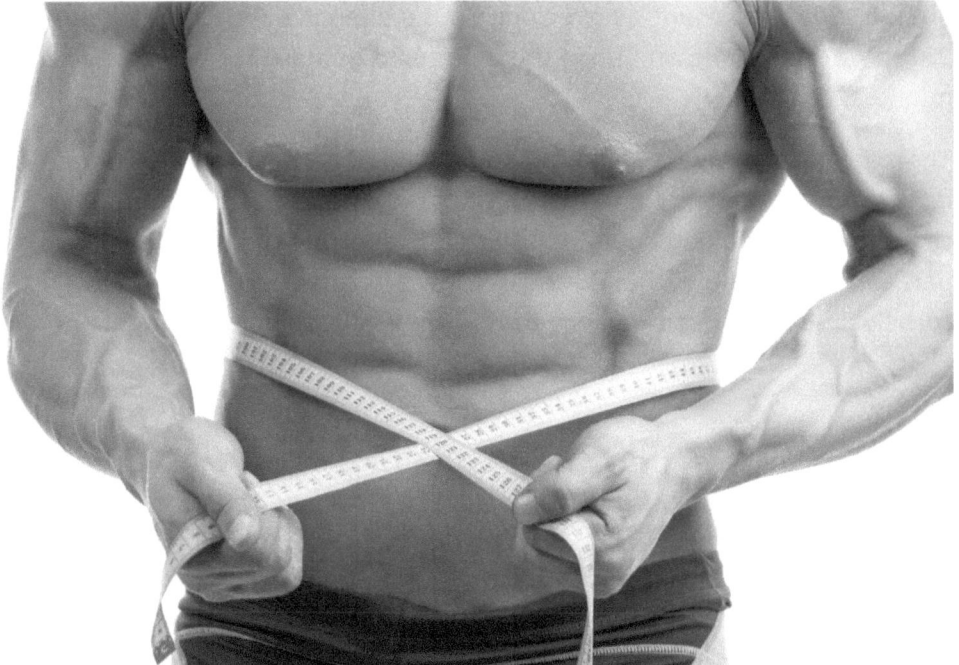

regularly throughout the day, at least 2 litres each day, more in hot weather and when you are working out. Little and often is best.

Tea and coffee do count, although not as much; count them as about half of the value of water.

FEEDING DURING TRAINING

would not expect anyone doing casual sport or any intense weight training to train with maximum intensity for longer than an hour, but it is important to know how to feed should you get involved in any endurance sessions or endurance training that last longer than that. If you are training or competing over the hour mark, taking in plenty of fluid and extra carbs will almost certainly help keep you going longer. Under an hour, and all you will need is a water bottle to sip at. I am amazed at how many trainers I see training at low intensity, with big breaks between sets, eating bars and drinking Lucozade. This is probably turning their healthy pursuit into another chance to stuff themselves and justify the need. You can work out very hard and with much intensity for an hour without needing to consume those often high-calorie sports bars and drinks as you train. Talking and lingering in a big training group for over an hour does not count as over one hour's exercise. C'mon guys, get real But for those of you who push the limits and go hard for over sixty minutes, read on.

The science says that consuming some kind of carbs during a workout lasting more than sixty minutes can help you keep going longer. The carbs keep your blood sugar levels steady and fuel the muscles, particularly when glycogen levels get low after the one-hour mark. The carbs will not convert to glycogen, but they will keep you going longer.

HOW MUCH

The science indicates that that between 30 and 60 g of carbs for each hour of exercise is ideal. That is about 120–240 cals per hour. More than that will not increase the benefits, as the muscles can't take up any more than that per hour from the bloodstream. How do you do it?

• Start consuming carbs early in your workout, ideally during the first thirty minutes, as it takes about thirty minutes for the carbs to be taken up. Waiting for an hour or until you feel tired would be too long.

• Choose fast-burning carbs with a high or moderate GI. You need to get them into the bloodstream fast. Little and often is the best feeding plan. Also, choose low-fat carb options, as fat slows the digestion process.

• If you are trying to lose fat, don't have extra carbs during your workout Your pace will slow, performance will suffer, and you will also run the risk of losing muscle. Bodybuilders losing fat before a contest generally accep that they will lose some muscle in the act of losing fat and looking for tha

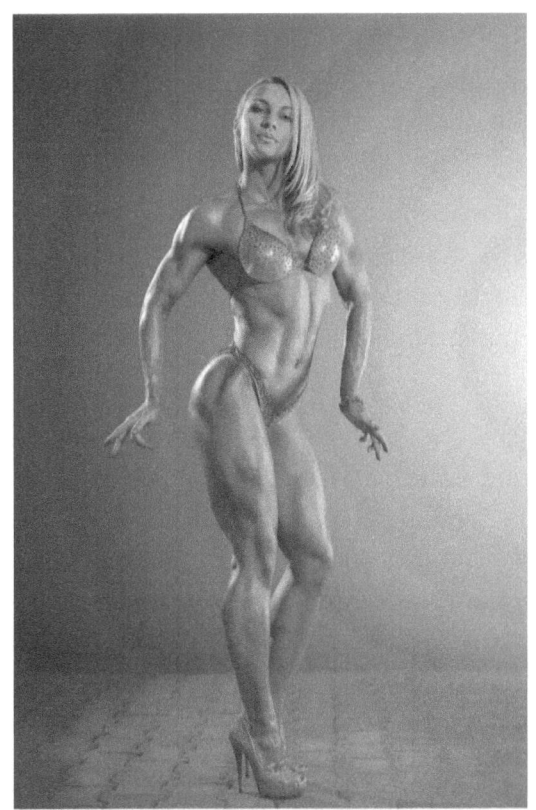

ripped appearance. Losing fat more gradually can minimise the muscle loss. But if your goal is extremely low body-fat levels, you will have to accept some muscle loss.

WHAT TO EAT

The foods need to be convenient and fast acting.

- Energy bar
- Cereal or breakfast bar
- Energy gels
- Raisins or sultanas • Bananas
- Low-fat biscuits

All should be consumed with plenty of water.

BOOSTING THE IMMUNE SYSTEM

Heavy, high-volume training results in increased levels of the stress hormones adrenaline and cortisol, which inhibit your immune system. What can you do to protect yourself?

- Eat enough calories to match your needs – eat more on training days.

- Prioritise immunity-boosting nutrients from your foods: vitamins A, C, and E, B6, zinc, iron, and magnesium. The best sources are fresh fruit, veg, whole grains, beans, lentils, nuts, and seeds.

- It is often wise to take a modest antioxidant supplement to boost your defences and reduce the risk of upper-respiratory infections. Avoid very strong supplements, as these are only to support your eating.

- Avoid training in a carb-depleted state.

- During long workouts of over one hour, take in 30–60 g of fast carbs an hour.

- Drink plenty of water.

- Echinacea for up to four weeks during hard training has been shown to boost the body's own production of immune cells and result in greater protection against progress-halting minor illnesses.

DRINKING WATER

If you don't drink enough water during exercise, or any at all, your blood begins to thicken, and your heart has to beat faster to circulate the thicker blood. This puts the body under undue stress that can be avoided just by sipping water during your workout and throughout the day. Dehydrated muscles are weaker. Losing 2 per cent of your body weight as sweat results in a 10–20 per cent drop in your aerobic capacity. Whatever you are doing, once you become even a little dehydrated it will be harder to keep up the same intensity, and you will be forced to drop your pace. Be in the habit of sipping water all day long and particularly when training. Feeling thirsty means you are already becoming dehydrated and it is too late to avoid a drop in intensity, but accept that and drink. Learn for the next time.

PERFORMANCE OR FAT LOSS

If you are looking to lose fat, drink just water during your training. Sports drinks may often provide more calories than you are burning off.

If your aim is to improve your fitness, strength, or performance in any way, and you are working out for extended periods, then sports drinks will help you keep going for longer.

FEEDING AFTER TRAINING

Once you have finished training, the important job of recovery takes place, or should take place. How you recover determines whether you improve or not. Training progress rests heavily on the recovery process. This is when you get bigger, stronger, and fitter.

What do you need to ensure you keep progressing in your intense training and to help you avoid wasting your time in the gym?

• Fluids: Replace the fluids lost through exercise. This is where your new habit of sipping water all day helps. The science says that during a workout you need to drink 750 ml for every half kg of body weight lost during your workout. Personally, I have never weighed myself and measured my water intake. I find just sipping water keeps your levels within optimum ranges.

• Electrolytes: If you sweat profusely and work out for a long time, you may lose electrolytes. Depending on the level of sweating, you may need to consume a sports drink. And if you are an endurance athlete or doing heavy cardio sessions, you will need more *than* someone doing an average weights workout.

• Carbs: These are crucial to recovery. There is a two-hour window after exercise when your body converts carbs into glycogen one and a half times faster than normal. If you work out regularly, speedy recovery is vital. We recommend clients have a carb/protein recovery shake immediately upon finishing training and another feed before the two hours have elapsed, to make full use of the faster conversion window. Get the recovery process underway ASAP.

• Protein: Added protein aids recovery much better than just carbs, particularly for intense muscle workouts with intense training. The protein boosts glycogen storage by almost 40 per cent, adding to the benefits of the faster muscle repair and growth in weight trainers. The science says that the combination of protein and carbs stimulates insulin release, which encourages the muscle cells to take up glucose and amino acids faster from the bloodstream.

• Antioxidants: One of the factors leading to muscle soreness is the build-up of free radicals, generated during exercise. Boost your body's natural defence against such free radicals by consuming plenty of foods rich in antioxidants. These include fruit, grains, veg and pulses.

POST-WORKOUT FEEDS

You will find that often you have no appetite post workout. Liquid meals can be the preferred option immediately after training. The ideal snack should contain carbs and protein. I have a few suggestions.

• Shake: There are many on the market. I take one to the gym in my kit bag; it's made up with skimmed milk, a protein blend, and carbs in the form of waxy maize and fine oats. The powders are often fortified with vitamins and minerals. A simple meal replacement shake will be perfect.

• Fruit and milk: A simple version of the above would be a pint of skimmed milk and a piece of fruit.

• Large carton of low-fat fruit yogurt.

• Smoothie made with skimmed milk and fruit of your choice

• Smoothie made with milk, yogurt, cottage cheese, and fruit

• Probiotic yogurt drink • Sports bar containing carbs and protein. These bars can be handy in your kit bag.

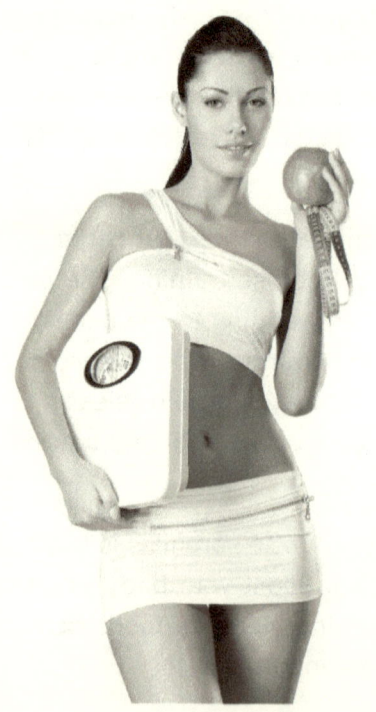

• Tuna, chicken, or cottage cheese sandwich made with whole-meal bread

• Porridge made with skimmed milk. This is always a good feed, as are other wholegrain cereals with milk.

• Jacket potato or sweet potato with tuna, chicken, or cottage cheese as the sandwich

It helps if you are organised and know where your next feed is coming from. We recommend, and indeed practise, consuming two of these feeds within the two-hour recovery window ollowing training. To stress the importance of nutrition, we also stress hat we would rather miss a workout than miss a feed. There is no point n tearing down muscle tissue if you have not planned to feed and recover ost-workout. I have met many trainers who are looking for the secret to heir progress or lack of it in new training methods, when nine times out f ten the answer is to be found outside of the gym, in the way they feed he body.

know many trainers are only able to work out late in the day and they vorry about eating too close to bedtime. Often they fast, because they elieve they will get fat if they sleep on food. The key is to eat well all day nd then not to overeat after training. There is an optimum amount. Vhen I used to work out evenings, I followed the same protocol. I had ny shake immediately after training, followed inside two hours by a ensible feed as per the list or similar. If we were on a fat-loss cycle, we vould have only protein for the second feed before bed, such as cottage heese or a protein blend shake (although not the most inspirational feed efore bed). At times of fat loss, the sacrifice has to be made – the neans to the end. And this leads us nicely on to the next section.

FEEDING FOR FAT LOSS

lo matter how much fat you need to lose, the principles of fat loss are he same: "Work out or move more and eat less." It's that simple. Food hoices become so vital. You become a product of your food choices. It is ard to get the balance right, and there is so much conflicting advice. hose in the food industry only care about profit and want to sell you as nuch food as possible. It is important rather than having a one-diet nentality and a separate normal eating pattern and mentality, to try to levelop habits that can be tweaked to give you the body that you want. ou will never gain too much fat and you will be in control.

his section is essential reading for anyone wanting to lose body fat. It jives the science on eating and exercising for fat loss, as well as tips that ave worked for us and many others.

he word diet normally entails a strict feeding (or lack of feeding) regime hat may cause some weight loss but makes you feel lethargic, weak, and hard done by, hindering your efforts in the gym. Worse than that, your body can end up storing instead of burning fat. Starvation mode is when your body fears starvation and goes into survival mode. The rate at which you burn fuel slows down. Your body adapts to survive on fewer calories, which means that when you resume normal eating, rather than maintaining a steady body weight, you're likely to put the weight back on. Added to that, to compensate for lower calorie intake, your body will start to break down muscle tissue to use for fuel, and you can end up losing your hard-earned muscle as well as fat. By far the best way to lose fat and keep it off is with regular exercise, plus a healthy and careful calorie intake, which includes a little-and-often feeding schedule of nutritious foods.

For the lowest health risk to the population, the science indicates that body fat levels between 18 and 25 per cent for women and 13 and18 per cent for men are optimum. However, lower body-fat levels are advantageous to performance in many sports, and levels in the region of

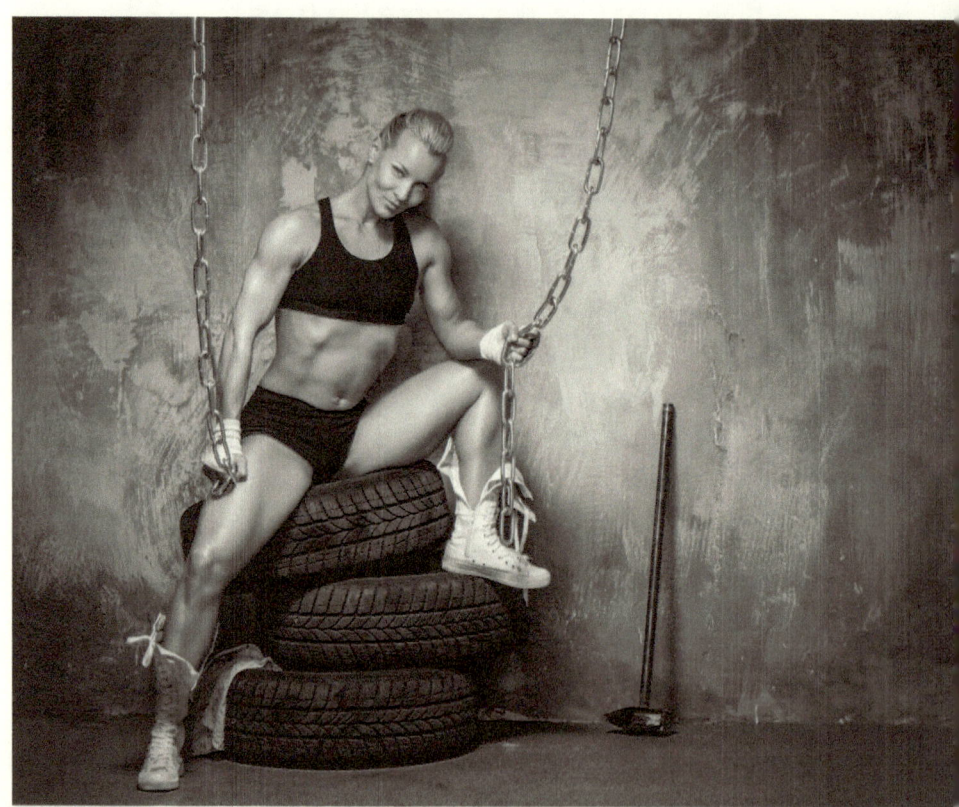

10–18 per cent in women and 5–10 per cent in men are common amongst elite athletes. Add to that the media and consumer industries' featuring of lower-body-fat men and women as the norm, and you have a false and often Photo-shopped ideal created to which all others aspire. The ideal created by these influences seems to be the lower the better.

ABOUT CALORIES

The only way to lose fat is to take in fewer calories than your body needs for basic functions and daily activity. Excess calories are stored as fat. It is that simple. Any "miracle diet" out there will only be effective if it is based on attaining a calorie deficit, through more exercise (moving more) and less food (feeding less).

One pound of fat equals 3,500 cal. If you eat that many calories over your needs for the day, then you will be a pound heavier. If you eat that many calories less than your needs, then you will lose a pound.

You may have noticed that 3,500 cals divided by 7 days = 500 cal. For a weight loss of a pound per week, you need to produce a 500 cals deficit. This is a sensible amount. With this in mind, if you cut your calories by 350 per day and increase your motion to burn an extra 150 per day, you can comfortably arrive at a 1-lb-per-week fat loss.

Experts agree that 1–2 lb per week is a healthy and effective rate of weight loss. Any amount over this probably means you are losing muscle (living tissue).

ABOUT METABOLISM

The metabolic rate is the rate your body converts the food you eat into energy, the rate your body burns calories for energy. Your basal metabolic rate (BMR) is the rate at which you burn calories on basic body functions, such as breathing, circulating blood, and maintaining body temperature. It does account for a major share of the calories you expend daily. To generalise, BMR uses 11 cals per pound of a woman's body weight and 12 cals per pound of a man's body weight. A 10-stone woman (140 lb) burns roughly 1,540 cals daily just to run her body. A 15-stone man (210 lb) burns roughly 2,520 cals daily just to run his body. This is

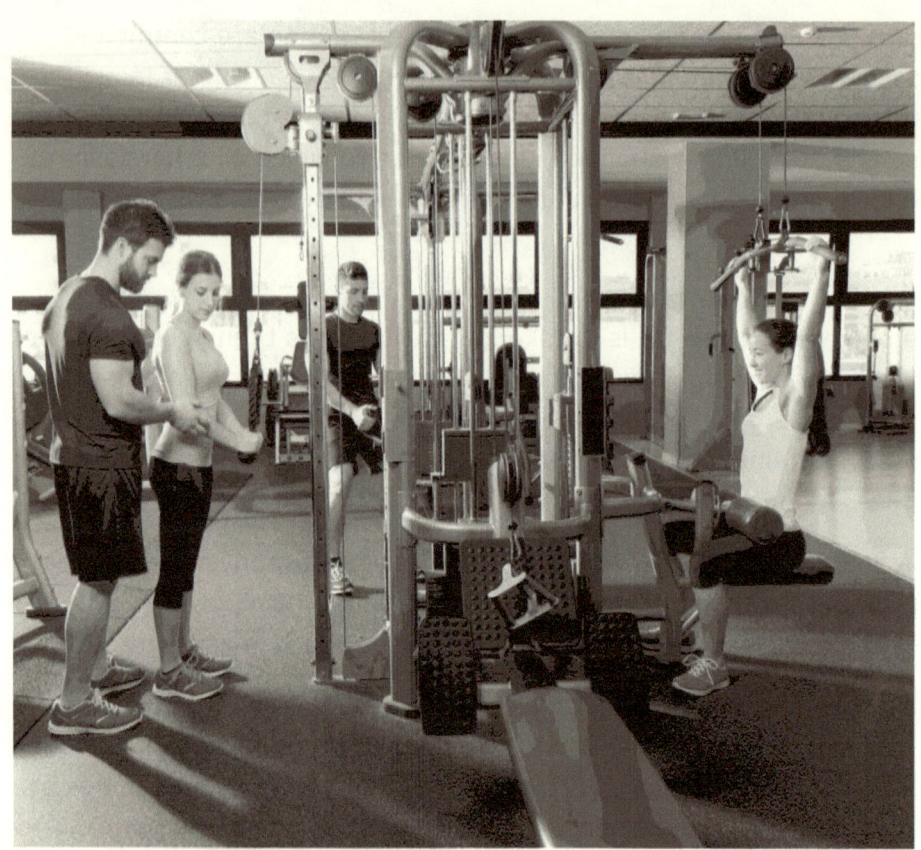

the rate without any physical activity at all. There is a catch: your BMR depends on the percentage of lean muscle tissue in your body. Muscle cells are many (8) times more metabolically active than fat cells, so the more muscle you have, the higher your BMR. As you can see, the figures above may vary over or under, depending on the composition of your body.

The safest way to increase your metabolic rate is with exercise. The harder you work, the faster your metabolic rate becomes. This increase continues after exercise, as your body burns extra calories to replenish its used stores of energy and repair muscle tissue. The more intense the training, the greater the calorie burn is afterwards. Intense weight workouts raise your metabolic rate for up five hours afterwards. Less intense aerobic workouts may burn on for less than an hour. Weight training is perfect for igniting your metabolism. To increase your metabolic rate more permanently, you have to increase your lean body tissue. Adding 2.2 lb (1 kg) of muscle is estimated to burn an extra 65 cals a day. So the more muscle you have, the easier it becomes to stay lean.

Unless you exercise regularly, you'll lose 0.25 kg (½ lb) of muscle every year after your late twenties or early thirties. From the paragraph above, you can see that as you lose muscle, you burn fewer calories – you get fatter quicker. The BMR drops about 2% each decade. Weight gain is then made worse by people cutting back on activity. Often they subscribe to the stereotypical view of getting older; they accept how one should be as one gets older.

To maintain your physique and body-fat levels, you would have to increase your calorie burn by 2 per cent or eat 2 per cent fewer calories. It's simple, really. If you needed 2500 calories when you were thirty, and you kept your calories in and out the same as you aged, that would amount to a 50-calorie surplus every day. Over 365 days, that is equal to 18,250 surplus calories, or a weight gain of 2.6 kg (5 lb). This is not something you would want to accept for every year that passes after your late twenties.

Luckily, you can beat age-related muscle loss with weight training; just two sessions per week can make the difference to your metabolism and your physique. Use it or lose it.

ABOUT TRAINING FOR FAT LOSS

The science says three cardio and two weights sessions per week are ideal. In reality, there lots of ways of splitting up your training to fit even the busiest schedules. A good plan is to alternate day weight sessions and cardio sessions. Be active every day.

We build our cardio into our lives and rarely perform cardio at a gym. We do this by daily walking the dogs at least 5 miles, by biking, and at times by doing a little stadium running, lunging, and jumping at a local cricket ground. The walking and biking is built into our lives. We decided to get rid of the car a couple of years ago. However, you don't need to get rid of your car to walk and bike every day, although having no car does make it an easier choice or no choice. The Great Body Bible does cover some training options, and any good personal trainer should be full of creative routines and splits for you, to prevent boredom. If your training and activity are well planned, you will be a walking calorie-burning furnace. The best antidote for boredom is seeing progress. Commit fully, and you will see the results.

Whether you are male or female, building muscle will make your body burn more calories daily, and the after-burn from your regular intense workouts will keep you revved up and heading in the right direction. The most effective strategy for building/ toning muscle and burning body fat simultaneously is high-intensity weight training. This doesn't mean lifting as much as you can but, rather, working each body part with a minimum of six sets and up to twelve sets, using a weight that you can only lift for between 8–12 reps (repetitions). The rest periods between sets are thirty seconds, maybe going up to a minute for heavy body-part exercises, such as leg and back work.

I have dealt with cardio in the paragraph above. I will now deal with the science or recommended amounts and methods. Twenty to forty minutes, three to five times per week is recommended.

Being aerobically fit increases your body's ability to burn fat. You will get aerobic fitness from your weights workouts if you are fast, with short rest periods, and your heart rate stays elevated throughout your workouts.

Don't overdo the cardio; the science shows that after about sixty to ninety minutes of aerobic activity, the body begins to break down and use muscle tissue as fuel. If you are restricting calories, this happens even earlier in your workout. Losing muscle means a lower BMR, so you won't burn as many calories.

The type of exercise that qualifies for cardio is any that uses large muscle groups with relatively low intensity, so it can be kept up for between twenty to forty minutes, with your heart rate in a set target range – aptly named your target heart range. Running, using cross trainers or cycles, fast walking, rowing, stepping, swimming, and even some group exercise classes – you can participate in any or all of these or find something I failed to mention. The important thing is the duration and time spent in your target heart range. If you are alternating with training with weights, is wise not to use too much resistance, as you may prevent your recovery from the training the day before.

The harder you work, the greater the calorie burn. However, remember that you may be recovering from your weight workout the day before. Active recovery is fine, but don't increase resistance and hamper your progress. For example, don't use too high a resistance on a rower the day after an arm workout or have the bike on a high level the day after working the legs. You get the picture – use some common sense.

TARGET HEART RANGE

As a guide, you should be working at about 60–85 per cent of your maximum heart rate (MHR). To get an idea of what this is for you, subtract your age from 220 and multiply by .6 and .85. I will give an example of a 40-year-old trainer:

As a guide you should be working at about 60-85% of you maximum heart rate (MHR). To get an idea of what this is for you, subtract your age from 220 and multiply by .6 and .85. I will give an example of a 40 year old trainer:

$$220 - 40 = 180$$

$$180 \times 0.6 = 108$$

$$180 \times 0.85 = 153$$

This trainer's target heart range is between 108 and 153 beats per minute (BPM). The higher in the range the trainer works, the fitter he will become. Above that level, and he may tap into the recovery from the previous day's weights workout, for little or no added advantage. Working higher may reduce the effectiveness of the fat burning.

WEIGHTS OR CARDIO?

What type of workout boosts your metabolic rate more, weights or cardio?

The science indicates when comparing an hour of each that both burned a similar amount of calories. However, the biggest difference occurred during the first two hours after exercise, with the weights workout increasing the metabolic rate much more. What's more, with the weights workout, the metabolic rate stayed higher than normal for up to fourteen hours afterwards. This proves that weights workouts are the best way to boost metabolism and burn more calories in the long term.

EARLY MORNING WORKOUTS

For fat loss, the best time to exercise is early morning, before eating, when insulin levels are at their lowest and glucagon levels are at their highest. (Glucagon promotes the breakdown of glycogen into glucose. This facilitates the process whereby fat leaves your fat cells and goes to the muscles, where it is burned as fuel.) You won't burn more calories, but the calories you will burn will be a higher percentage of fat calories. This will lead to speedier fat loss over a number of weeks or months. However, performance will suffer, and to perform better it is still advisable to feed pre-workout as discussed earlier. The resulting rise in blood-glucose levels slows the rate of stored glycogen depletion, enabling you to exercise harder and longer. A personal example of how this can work is that I walk the dogs for at least a few miles every morning.

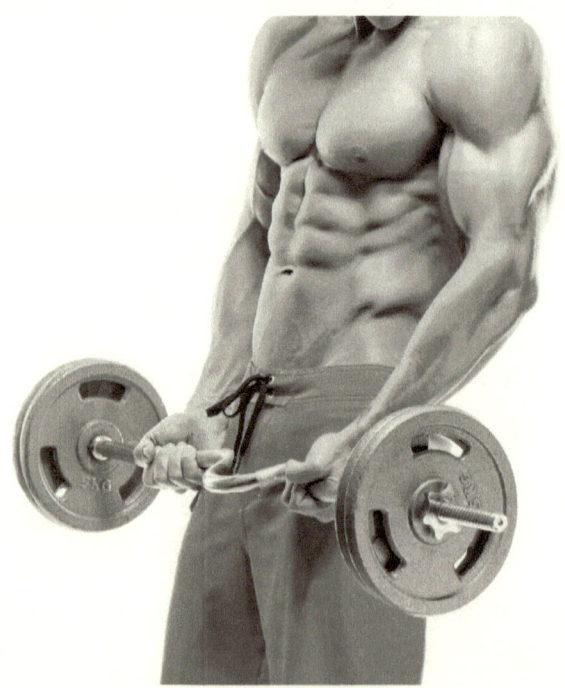

Performance on my walk is not paramount. There are no dog-walking contests in my area. This allows me to walk on an empty stomach, burning fat. After walking the dogs at 4.30 a.m., I also travel to the gym on my bike for 6 a.m. some mornings to train clients. The same applies here; I also do this on an empty stomach. I have always fed by between 7 a.m. and 8 a.m. Later in the day at the gym (11 a.m.), when it becomes more important to perform, I make sure I am well fed. That is an example of how you can use fat burning to your advantage.

FEEDING FOR FAT LOSS

How many calories should you be eating? There are two method of determining this.

This method is for people who are already on a fairly low-calorie intake. Reducing calories by 15 per cent will minimise the drop in your metabolic rate that can occur when you reduce calories. Record your calorie intake for seven days. Be as accurate as possible, and include anything with a calorific value. I have known people not to include drinks. This list is meant to be all inclusive. You will only hamper your own progress by falsifying the information. I know it sounds obvious, but I have seen people worrying so much about their list looking good – whatever that may be in this context – that it little resembles reality. Use food tables, the Internet, and food labels to work it all out. The next step is to add the seven days together and then divide by seven to get a daily average. Then just subtract 15 per cent from that number (x 0.85), this will be your new daily intake to start losing fat.

Calculating your calorie requirements.

Estimate your basal metabolic rate (BMR).

Women: BMR = weight in kg's x 2 x 11(or weight in lb's x 11)

Men: BMR = weight in kg's x 2 x 12 (or weight in lb's x 12)

An example for 60kg man BMR = 60 X 2 X 12 = 1440 cals

Next estimate activity level:

Inactive or sedentary: BMR X 20%

Fairly active (walk or exercise 1-2 times per week): BMR X 30%

Moderately active (exercise 2/3 times per week): BMR X 40%

Active (exercise hard more than 3 times per week): BMR X 50%

Very active (exercise hard daily): BMR X 70%

For our moderately active 60kg man 1440 x 40% = 576

Add the two together to work out your daily calorie needs. For our moderately active 60-kg man it would be 1440 (BMR) + 576 (activity) = 2016 cal.

That is the amount of calories our man needs to maintain his weight if he is of an average body composition. If he was more muscular than average, you would add 150 cals to this amount to allow for his higher metabolic rate.

Remember that to lose ½ kg (1 lb) you have to create a 3,500 cals deficit. As discussed previously, to lose you need to subtract 350 cals from your daily amount and increase your activity each day to burn 150 cal.

KEEP A JOURNAL

This is the part when I tell you to write down everything that you eat. That is right, but a journal is so much more than that. Write down your feeds and times in detail. Also write down your activity sessions and anything worthy of the name exercise. Writing this down can spur you on to get as much in the activity column as possible, at least something active every day. I find that it also helps to vent your feelings about all that is happening and to tweak all that is too uncomfortable to ever become a new habit or regular behaviour. A journal also helps when you are next looking to lose fat. You will see what worked and what didn't and it will remind you of much that will have slipped your mind once you have reached your fat-loss goals.

INTERPRET THE ISSUES

Once you see them written down, you will see that some of your food choices are definite mistakes if you are serious about dropping fat. Work out which foods you need to increase or reduce. Work out when you are strong and motivated and when you are having issues sticking to your plan, and adapt accordingly. Fat is high calorie, and most often the culprits are snacks, biscuits, crisps, puddings, ice cream, cakes, and chocolate bars. Get real – get rid!

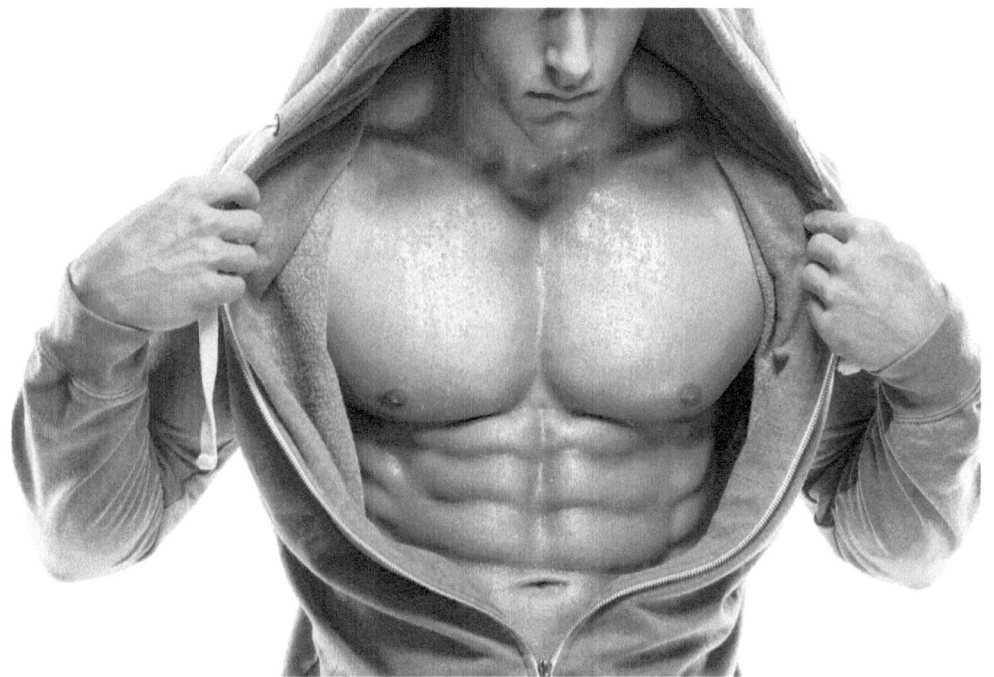

SLOW BURN

Oats, beans, lentils, veg, and fruit are slow burning and essential. Drop white bread, soft drinks, and sugary cereals. Eating carbs with protein or essential fatty acids balances blood-sugar levels better than eating carbs alone. This will have less effect on insulin, the hormone that drives fat into your fat cells. Slow-burn foods improve appetite regulation and increase feelings of fullness. Eat slowly to allow your mind to catch up with your body in feeling full.

FAT-LOSS COMMON SENSE

Eat little and often. By spreading your feeds through the day, as four, six, or even more (depending on weight) small feeds rather than two or three big feeds, you will avoid those blood-sugar highs and lows and the resulting insulin surges. Insulin is an extremely powerful anabolic hormone that drives glucose from the bloodstream into the muscle cells and, here is the catch, when there's too much glucose around, into your fat cells, too. Your goal should be to keep your blood-glucose and insulin levels stable at levels that never allow for that extra glucose to be stored as fat. The reduced chances of fat storage and the added benefit of your metabolism being revved all day makes this a wise tactic for fat-loss now and maybe a habit worth developing for life. Throw out the three meals per day conditioning and join the little and often (every two or three hours) brigade. You can imagine how bad for your fat levels the starters-main course-and desert mentality is. The only beneficiaries of that antiquated behaviour are the food sellers. Old habits die hard, but die they must in the name of your health and physique.

Eating the right foods is common sense, as fat will make you fatter than protein or carbs. Fat is already close in its makeup to the form it needs to be in for fat storage. To metabolise fat, the body requires just 3 cals for every 100 cals that you eat. This leaves 97 to be stored in your fat cells. Carbs require 10–15 cals, leaving 85–90 to be stored, whereas protein requires an amazing 20 cals to use it, leaving 80. So it is easy to see that protein and carbs are your best bets if you want to increase your metabolic rate and reduce the amount of excess available to be stored as fat. You might be thinking all of this is only making a negligible difference, but over time and with the common-sense tips being many, the gain is massive. All the little changes add up to one big change in your health and physique.

The science shows that limiting your food choices helps with fat loss. Why? It's because, when faced with a bigger choice, you will eat more total calories. A bit of this and a bit of that ads up to more than if you limit your choice by knowing what you are going to eat. When you shop, limit the variety of your shop, thereby limiting your choices and the temptation to overindulge. Simplify your feeds. I am smiling as I type

his, because I have had two
eeds in the first few hours of
his morning, and both have
•een porridge (oatmeal) with
kimmed milk. It does the job for
ne. If you have a problem food,
on't buy it! When the urge hits,
: will pass without you
abotaging your fat-loss efforts.

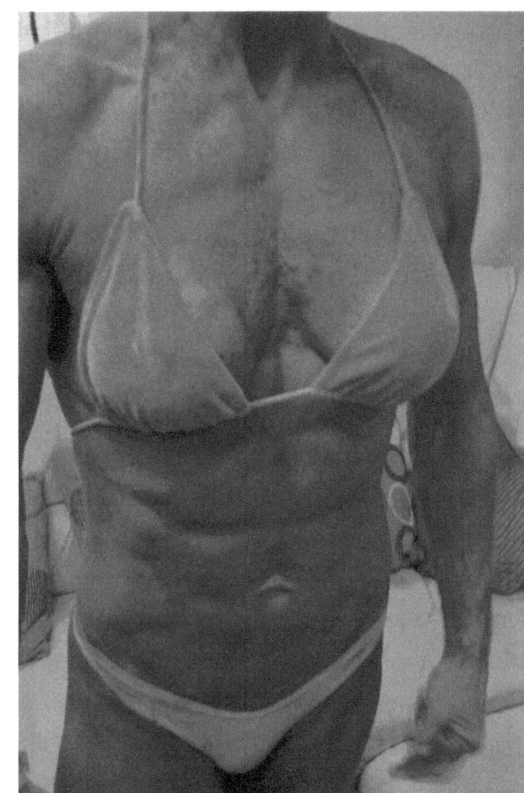

ortion control can be a blessing
ι the battle for fat loss. At first
ou may have to measure and
veigh your foods, but eventually
ou will automatically know how
nuch and in which bowl. Having
arge portions just means
vereating. Little and often, not
•ig and often, is the way to go.
nother strategy we use,
•articularly when getting ready for a show, is to use small plates for
very feed. The temptation to overfill the plates is then taken away, and
here is the added psychological benefit of seeing your plate amply filled
s opposed to a large plate being empty and "poor you" feeling starved
nd hard done to.

'ou don't have to skip your favourite foods altogether. You are calorie
ounting, so as long as they fit into your total plan, you can include them.
ndulge occasionally. A little of what you fancy may do you good, but
emember that too much will make you fat and may eventually kill you.

ncrease your protein when you reduce your calories. The need for
•rotein increases to prevent a loss of muscle, and to maintain your
netabolic rate, as seen above, protein takes 20 cals to metabolise 100.
'hat is a good boost to your metabolism. The science shows that protein
akes the edge off your appetite more than carbs or fat. If you don't have
nough protein, you may find yourself still hungry after you've eaten. Eat
 fist-sized portion at least with each feed.

A good feed in the morning gets your metabolism off to the right start and allows you the whole day to burn those calories. Your body is more insulin sensitive in the morning and less in the evening as your cortisol levels go up. In real terms this means that you can handle carbs more efficiently in the morning than in the evening. The carbs are more likely to be used for fuelling your daily activity, whereas later in the day there i a greater chance they will be stored as fat. The science shows that not feeding well in the morning makes you more likely to snack and overindulge at lunch time. Dieters who ate a high-fibre breakfast lost more weight than those who didn't eat breakfast.

There is a habit in society of getting up late, having a sketchy breakfast, being busy all day, with a grabbing-food attitude, and then eating a large meal in the evening. This has got to change. It's much better to eat a smaller meal of mainly protein and veg before going to bed. Avoid eating for the two hours prior to retiring. Close to bedtime, bodybuilders may have a protein only shake or a tub of plain cottage cheese to aid the recovery and growth process and to compliment growth hormone release during sleep. Eating the bulk of your calories in the evening, when you are inactive, increases the chances of storing them as body fat.

Appetite is often confused as real hunger. The food industry aims at marketing to your appetite to sell their product. Appetite is produced by external stimuli, such as the sight or smell of food, boredom, or the television advertising you stare at every evening. Genuine hunger is produced internally when your blood sugar levels begin to fall. The difference is that appetite goes away if you are distracted away from the external stimulus. Genuine hunger does not. Try this! Next time you feel the urge to eat, go for a walk, take a bath, or do something to distract yourself. If you are still hungry, then you need to eat. Sadly, we are conditioned to feed through appetite, and that is why so many people in our society are obese.

All fats are not created equal. In your efforts to exclude fat from your diet, make sure you keep in your healthy fats. Oily fish, avocados, nuts, olives, and seeds in moderation can help you burn body fat more efficiently, improve aerobic capacity, and boost your immunity.

Alcohol contains 7 cals per gram. Alcohol calories can't be stored and have to be used as they are consumed, which means other calories are stored as fat instead. If you have a drink, include the calories in your total. But wise up – if you are wanting to lose fat, ditch the alcohol and drink water.

Thirst and hunger feelings are generated simultaneously by the brain. You may be thirsty and assume that you are hungry, so you feed instead of drinking water. When you feel peckish, have a drink of water and wait for fifteen minutes to see if you still feel hungry.

It is always wiser and a calorie saving to eat the fruit as opposed to drinking the fruit juice or, for that matter, eating the dried fruit. Dried fruit and juice are higher in sugar. Go for the real-fruit option, and drink water.

Food labels can be very misleading. "Reduced fat" or "light" often means more sugar. Check the calorie count on the label, and don't be fooled.

One of the secrets to eating healthier or eating for fat loss is not to have the high calorie options in your home. If you go shopping when you are hungry, you are more likely to fill up your trolley with high-calorie foods. Write your shopping list before you go to shop. Then you will avoid making unplanned purchases of unhealthy foods. Shopping with a list, you are less likely to succumb to appetite and make impulsive food choices. Supermarkets are in the business of selling you as much as they can. You need to be armed against their promotions and profit-mongering and be able to defend your health and your physique.

A good way of saving calories is to replace half of your starchy carbs, such as bread, potatoes, and pasta, with vegetables, such as carrots, green beans, and cauliflower.

You will be able to find an excuse for all bad eating habits. Stop using excuses. Take healthy foods with you wherever you go. Be prepared. If you eat when you watch television, stop watching television. You may actually do something active instead. Just think of the brain cells you will reactivate by not sitting in a trance in front of the television. You may be able to tell that we have no television. You will read later about the decision to completely remove the television from our lives. I will just leave it at that for now.

Be organised. Carry the food you need with you. Healthy snacks, shakes, or even made-up calorie-counted meals. Don't get caught not having the choice to eat as you planned. Vending machines and snack-food counters are not fat-loss friendly.

Just eat one course. Three or more courses are archaic and will always result in fat storage – always.

Back to my favourite subject. The science indicates that watching television makes you eat more. People watching television for a few hours daily consume a third more calories. This is because they can sit in a trance and nibble or stuff food, whilst barely moving compared against others who actually have a life.

XXI. Once you decide on your strategy for fat loss and know the foods that are going to feature heavily, make sure you are well stocked. This will make your fat-loss programme easy. I am going to make you all raise

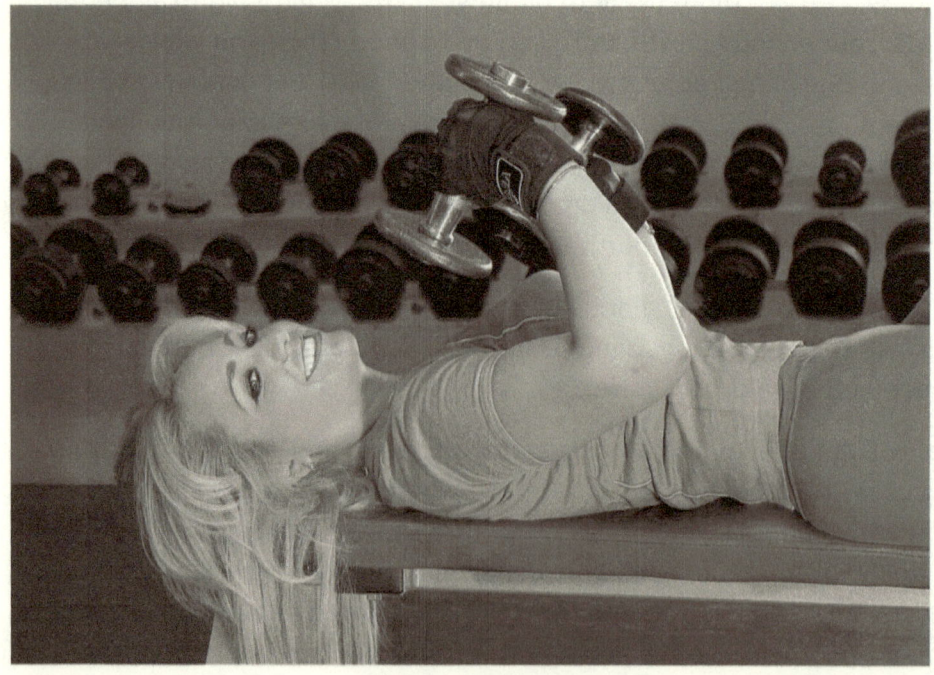

your eyebrows now by using a cliché: "Fail to plan, plan to fail." Be organised. It works.

FEEDING FOR THE GYM

If you are using the gym, you are in all probability aiming to change your body shape for whatever you have in mind. It may be you are lifting weights to get stronger, build muscle, or improve your definition (lose fat), all of which will result in a different body. You are going to need a smart eating plan. Correct feeding will give you the results you demand much quicker or even be the difference between making progress or hitting an early training plateau and stagnating. Maybe you are a hard gainer – you are lean and find it hard to gain muscle. Maybe you seem to get fat without muscle and need better definition, which means muscle without much fat to cover it. Either way, the answer lies in nutrition and what you do away from the gym. You need to devise a feeding strategy that allows you to gain muscle without it being covered in a layer of unwanted fat.

The training is covered in detail below and in the demonstration videos on Youtube – The Fitness Wizards channel. However I will discuss now how to train for building muscle. Male or female. The short version.

TRAINING THE ACTIVE BODY

To build muscle, you need to combine training, feeding, and resting. The idea is to train with enough intensity to break down muscle proteins and cause very small (micro) tears in the muscle fibres. During the all-important rest period between workouts, with adequate food made available, new protein is added to the fibres, making the muscle stronger and denser. Not only does the resulting muscle burn more calories, but the muscle-building process also requires extra energy (calories), which your body can take from stored body fat. So you burn more calories while you build muscle. I will outline below some basics for training in the gym. There are literally dozens of effective training regimes out there. Some are good, and some are best left alone. The following is not the last word on working out, but it will take you to a very good standard and may be all you will ever need.

~ 46 ~

GYM TRAINING: COMMON SENSE

• Aim for 8–12 sets on large muscle groups, such as legs, chest, back, and shoulders and 3–6 sets on smaller muscle groups, such as biceps and triceps.

• The repetition range to be aimed for is between 6 and 12 reps. We prefer to be on the high side. The weight used should ensure you fail on the last set or at least that you couldn't do another rep in proper form even if you put your house on it.

• The rest period between sets should be 60–90 seconds or as long as it takes your partner to perform his or her set and adjust the weights. Take a slightly longer rest between body parts but not much longer.

• Multi-joint (compound) movements are the best for gaining strength and muscle size; these include squats, bench press, shoulder press, and leg press. These stimulate the largest muscle groups. It is a good idea to use at least two different exercise for each muscle group, and a split system can also work well for keeping intensity high.

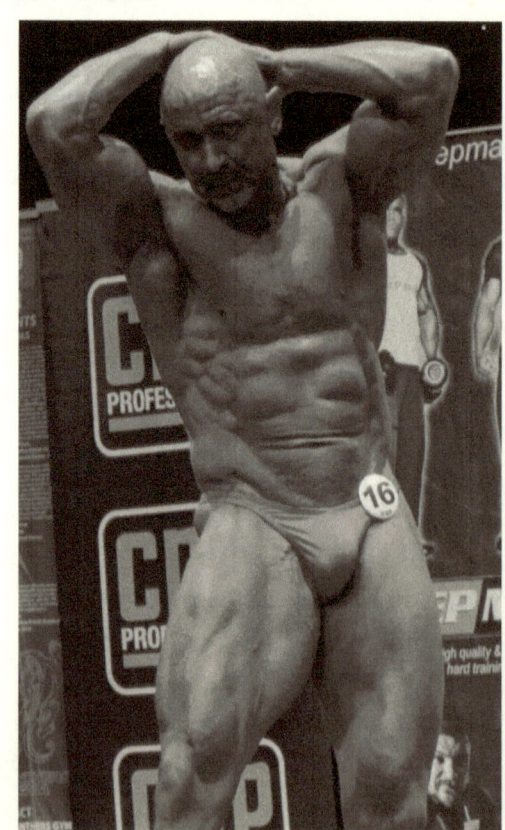

• Always train with proper form. Never sacrifice form for using more weight. You are cheating and will soon reach a plateau or get injured. Others are not as impressed as you think by your weight-lifting heroics, and even the novice trainer can spot cheating a mile off. Use a weight that allows a full range of movement with a tempo that is always under your muscle control. Using momentum will result in injury eventually. I remember being told by a mature trainer years ago that your tempo should enable you to pause the movement momentarily at any point in the exercise. That would be very strict form but still good advice.

Once you have gone past the beginner stage and have gained an element of confidence in the gym, there are some tried and trusted techniques to take you forward.

. Routines can be split up in all sorts of weird and wonderful ways. We like the straight upper body-lower body split. I won't list them all here but do have something quite amusing to relate. We trained at a gym where the gym experts were so busy and being listened to by others that on any given day almost everyone was doing the same body part, and all of that equipment would be busy all day. We just made sure we were never synchronised with the automatons, and we were able to have a free run at that gym, knowing what most of the others would be working on any given day. The point here is that there are many ways to split sessions, and variety is a valuable tool for shocking the body into new growth. Even funnier was the fact that leg days were either not in the split or nobody turned up for them. If you are new to the gym, you will find a high percentage of men who never train legs. Even something simple like doing the exercises in a different order will shake your routine up a little. There are no hard and fast rules.

I. Make your routines more intense by adding more reps, doing forced reps with a training partner, or doing partial reps where you complete as many full reps as possible and then just knock out half reps until you have had enough. Even increasing the weight and doing less reps, or cutting the rest between sets, or slowing down your rep tempo are other ways to up the intensity. We always try to adhere to the "time under tension" rule that says the way to increase intensity is through the total time the muscle is under extreme tension in each set. We use forced reps and supersets at our most intense times. We occasionally up the weight and drop the reps but are mindful of the weight lifted becoming the priority; this is not ideal for physique enhancement of any kind. An example of a superset for chest is a set of dumb-bell flyes followed by bench pressing with no rest between the two.

III. Increase your knowledge of exercises to enable you to use more variety. Every new variation stresses the muscle in a slightly different way. Be sure of what you are doing. I have seen many trainers interpreting something they have seen to use in the gym, and it is either totally unrecognisable or odd enough not to be of any use for their workouts – or maybe even dangerous. Be sure your form is right and tha you have mastered the move. The Great Body Bible has many ideas for adding variety to your workouts.

IV. Totally change your workout every month or so or if you are proficien and know many exercises for the body parts. Go to the gym with an idea of the body part you are going to work, and put the workout together ad lib. For instance, if you are due to train chest and back, keep in mind tha you need to do one lateral motion and one press for chest, and one row and one pull-down for back as a minimum. Then perform any variation that fulfils that criteria. This is an ideal strategy for a busy gym, as you can use what is available and not have to wait because you have to work in a set order. Be flexible. It is much more fun. Change will never halt your progress. Change will keep your body growing and off guard, with very few sticking points, as you will not allow them to set in.

V. A training partner can be a liability or an asset. You will need a common goal, and you will each need to have the other's progress as a priority. You will both have to be on time. It is a commitment. I have trained with women most of my training life, because the competition is much healthier. It's not about who can lift more, which stunts progress, but about how hard you train and encourage the others' progress. The energy has to be positive, and you have to be there for

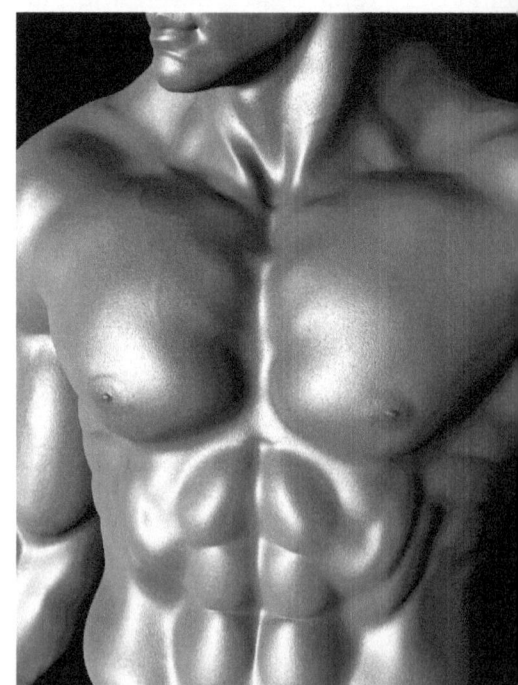

your partner for forced reps, negatives, and general encouragement. The time between your working set is all about them and the next set. There's no doing your set and then messing around until your turn comes around again. You have to participate the whole time, for them and yourself. You need to get to know them better than they know themselves in the gym. Advise and encourage them. Be their form guide, keep them honest with no lies to make them feel better if they are cheating.

VI. I have seen this regularly: a guy doing the worst bench press in the universe and his partner enthusing about how great it was. Cut the crap. The right choice of training partner is a win-win situation. The wrong choice can be a nightmare. I have seen partners who have become slaves to the dominant male and had no say in their workout's structure. Give and take is the order of the day. And an open mind to trying things that your partner may want to experiment with is a good thing. Such selflessness pays off, because that is where the golden nuggets of progress are discovered – in the places you would not have ventured without your guide. Keep your mind wide open. Find a good partner or train alone. Look out for worthy role models to emulate. Create high standards for yourself and your partner. Maybe at first you can just join in with other trainers who train alone; like any relationship, once you find a good chemistry and it feels right for both of you, you can make it a more regular arrangement. Be careful how you choose – I have been married to my training partner for thirty+ years!

BODY TYPES AND MUSCLE DEFINITION

To achieve a defined look when you are smooth (fat), you must drop body-fat levels; it is as simple as that. A "defined" look is not a special appearance, just well-developed muscle with low body fat. Many trainers believe that you have to train with lighter weights and higher reps to achieve a defined look. That is not true; that's another gym myth. That training can improve endurance, but it isn't the best way to burn fat. This has been covered previously.

The prime concern is to achieve the right calorie intake. Hard gainers (lean/skinny) will need to up the calories, whilst those looking to achieve definition (smooth/fat) may need to cut down the calories. How many calories do you require for the separate goals?

To gain good lean weight, the science states that increasing calories by 20 per cent should show results. In reality, men will need to add between 500 and 1000 cals a day to their usual intake. Women will need to add between 250 and 500 extra calories daily. Remember not to overdo the increase, as any surplus will be stored as fat. It is a common occurrence for novice trainers to be in such a hurry to "get big" to fit in that they eat freely and just get very fat. Be warned, as I have seen many good physiques ruined by this get-big mentality. Quality, not quantity, is the way to go. Patience is a vital ingredient to developing that eye-catching physique. Your weight should increase by no more than 0.25 and 0.5 kg (½–1 lb) per week, and even then there may be a period of fat loss needed after a weight-gain period. If your weight remains the same, you are not eating enough to support your training and growth. Don't be on the scales every day; once per week is enough.

To get more defined (drop body fat), adding extra cardio work and upping your overall activity level may be all you need to do. Walk more in general, and do three twenty- to forty-minute aerobic sessions per week. If you don't have too much to lose, this should do the trick nicely. However, if you are carrying more than 15 per cent (men) or 25 per cent (women) body fat, you almost certainly need a two-pronged attack of more activity and less calories. It is good to start to reduce your calories by about 15 per cent

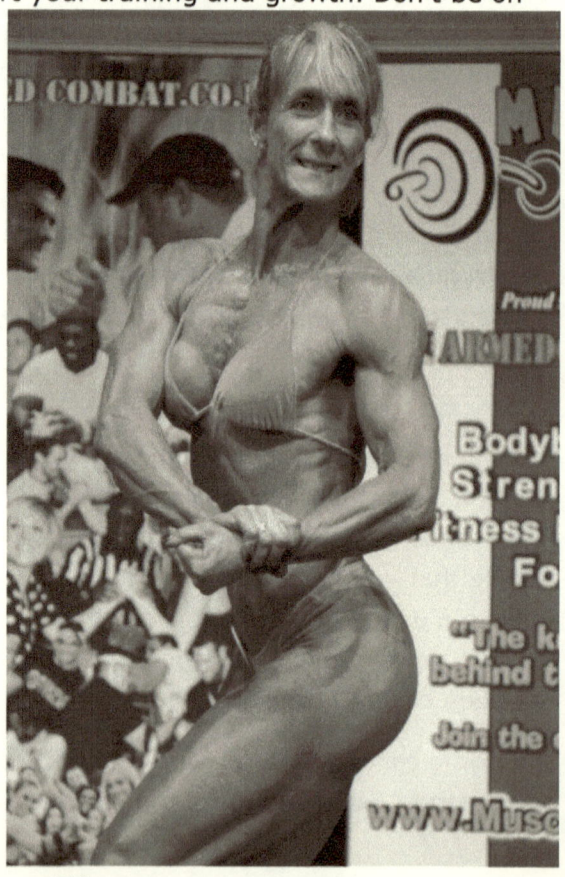

– that would amount to about 400 cals for men and 300 cals for women, depending on your body weight.

When cutting calories, remember not to be too impatient, as too low an intake will force your body to resist losing fat (starvation mode). We mentioned this in the fat loss section.

Body fat levels can be checked by someone skilled with skinfold callipers or by electrical-impedance equipment such as body composition scales. This will tell you how much of you is fat and how much of you is muscle. A skilled fitness professional will even be able to estimate your levels if they have much experience in working with clients of varying body compositions. Whilst this is useful to know occasionally, do not get hung up on scales and weights. It is good to use them for a guide, but I have seen a number on a scale totally change a happy person's mood; this was after a great session and good progress in the gym. If you are happy with what you see and are making good progress, never let a number on a machine control your feelings of well-being.

As I mentioned earlier, when attempting to gain weight, if you gain 3 kg of muscle and 1 kg of fat, you are going well. This is why it is better to cycle your diet and training goals into weight-gain and fat-loss cycles. If done properly, the overall result will be more muscle. Plus, it is great to vary your goals, diet, and sessions accordingly, preventing staleness or getting stuck in a physical rut.

However, if you gained 2 kg of fat and 2 kg of muscle in the same period, it would be wise to trim your carbs and overall calories. Being a little bit of a realist, in the field I see trainers trying to gain muscle, and the gain is more likely to be 6 kg of fat and 3 kg of muscle. For some reason, the urge to get big takes over, and fat becomes accepted or ignored in favour of a higher number on the scales – which means nothing if there is no quality to your physique! Have patience. Quality takes a little more time, but it is well worth the wait. Practise moderation in the land of plenty.

THE KEY TO MUSCLE GAIN: OPTIMUM PROTEIN INTAKE

After you have arrived at the correct calorific intake for your body size and shape, protein is the next most important part of your weight-training feeding plan. Amino acids (protein) are used by the body to repair the training damage. Without optimum protein as part of every feed, you can forget muscle growth. I use the word optimum (ideal) to mean that the right amount of protein is the key; the idea is not to eat massive amounts and hope for the best. Protein, whilst key, can easily

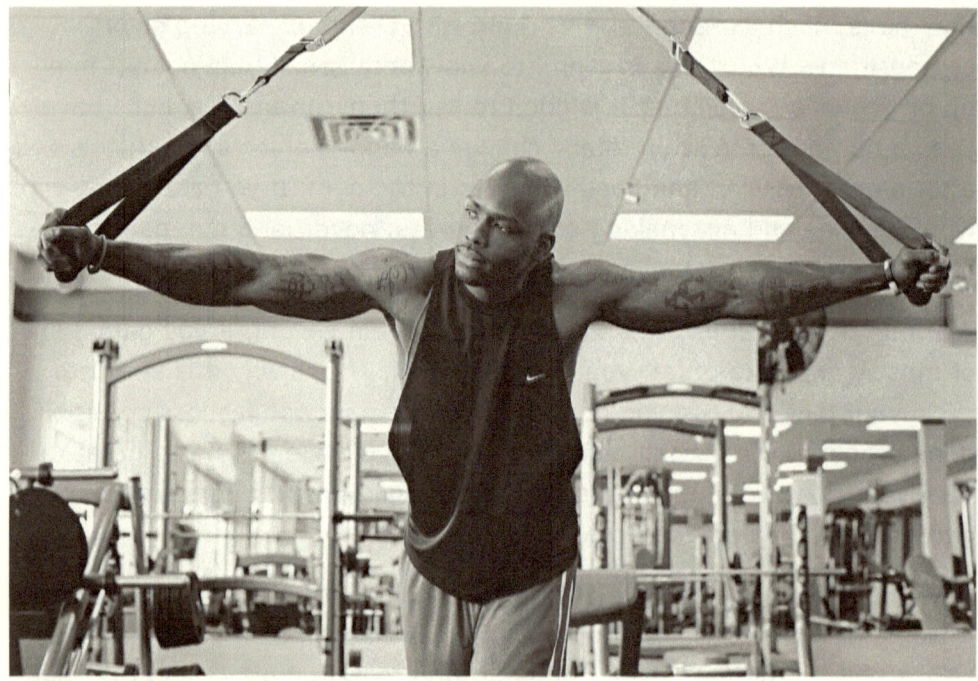

make you fat as excessive unused calories.

If you are pumping iron at least three times per week, the science says you will need between 1.4 and 1.8 g of protein per kg of body weight. If you weigh 70 kg, that is about 98–126 g daily. Bodybuilders may go as high as 2g per kg of body weight or even higher. Two things to remember are that they may be chemically enhanced, and they may be victims of the higher-protein-is-best sales philosophy of the bodybuilding supplement companies. Confused? You should be. I will add my thoughts on this matter.

feel that a moderate amount with every feed is the way to go. I have never been a greedy bodybuilder, and I weigh in at about 100 kg. I have been as heavy as 125kg, I have abs all the time, and I'm well into my fifties. I feel this is down to eating little and often and not eating too many carbs late in the day, my last feed being purely protein. For gaining weight, I add more feeds into my day. I have been as high as ten small late feeds per day. A shake is a feed, and the others might be porridge, chicken breast salad, fish salad, sweet potato, and a protein source. As you can see, all of my feeds are small and taper off in carbs later in the day. It works for me. Once you have a list of feeds that suit your tastes, it is an easy feeding system to stick to. I lose fat on six or seven strict feeds and gain on ten slightly less-strict feeds. Spreading protein across the whole day seems like good sense; if you are on a gaining regime, try beginning with six feeds and gauging your progress. Only add another feed when you feel the need. Begin with four solid feeds and two shakes (one post-workout with carbs and one bedtime, purely protein). I steer clear of large meals, and as for multi-course meals, they are for conformist robots and as outdated as the ark. If you want a physique to be proud of, learn to graze healthily. An example would be for 3,000 cals per day, six feeds every two to three hours, with an average of 500 cals each feed. Operate with that system, and gauge your weight depending on your goals. If you want to gain and are staying the same, just add another feed daily and so on. Feeds can fluctuate between 700 cals and 300 cal. There's no absolute rule; just use good reason (common sense). If you try to go too low on any feed you will overcompensate on later feeds. Stick to your plan, and adjust as needed.

PROTEIN SUPPLEMENTS

Protein supplements are food. Taking protein supplements won't give you bigger gains than what you might call normal food, but they can be a hell of a lot more convenient. Moreover, when you are feeding regularly, it can be nice just to have a shake, rather than having to plan a feed that might not even rival that simple shake for nutritional content. They are a viable option. Your goal is to have protein with every feed. It is up to you how you do that. I love to use high-protein foods and "normal" foods. The biggest drawback would be the cost. If you can afford it, the convenience is worth it. I have high-protein bread, protein and carb powders; ready meals (macronutrient counted), and I will use anything that I consider cost effective and that makes feeding easier and more varied. I prepare food for clients, and I often use specialist foods. If we use these regularly, they will one day be considered normal! Protein powder can be added to other foods, such as porridge, to make them higher in protein. You would be wise not to rule anything out of your options for feeds. You will also be amazed at the range of high-protein products becoming available as demand increases. As ever, keep an open mind.

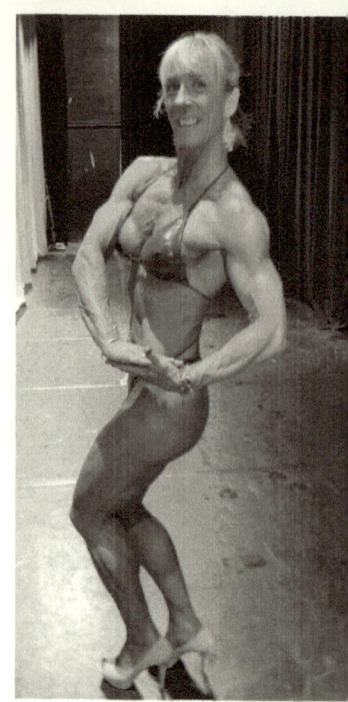

BEST FUEL: CARBS

The major fuel you use for lifting weights is carbohydrates. In an intense workout you may deplete up to half of your glycogen (stored carbs) reserves in your muscles. To restock, you must eat carbs. Without them you will feel weak and not be able to deliver the intensity needed to stimulate muscle growth. With full glycogen stores, your body can hold onto protein to build muscle. Without adequate glycogen, valuable protein is used for fuel and not for building muscle. You will end up smaller, not bigger.

Carbs also raise insulin levels. Insulin is an anabolic hormone, driving protein and carbs into the muscle cells to facilitate repair and growth. You need the right amount; otherwise insulin drives the surplus into the fat cells. What is the optimum (ideal)? Once again, you can have too much of a good thing. How much is enough?

If you are pumping iron three to five times per week, aim to have 5–7 g of carbs per kg of body weight per day. Your amount of fuel does ultimately depend on your activity levels, as you would expect with a fuel source. If you are a hard gainer (lean/skinny), you are sure you are getting enough protein, and you are stuck with your progress, increase your carbs by 50 g per day for a few days and then another 50 g, until you start to grow again.

If you are a hard gainer, spread your carbs throughout the day. Otherwise, targeting your fuel around your activity works best. Taper off toward bedtime and the long period of inactivity. Protein only should form the last feed of the day. The most important time is directly after exercise and again within two hours. This promotes faster glycogen uptake as well as higher levels of growth hormone.

CONCLUSION

Outlined here in this book are the basics for good nutritional health. You will come across many diets and feeding plans that do not follow these rules. The truth is that the human body doesn't really change that much, and what you have here are the facts, the basics. These are things that will work every time.

Are there any secret diets or shortcuts? If something seems too good to be true, it generally is. There are many looking for profits in the diet industry. To achieve these, they need to continually market new products to the often-desperate public. The basics, when done right, give the results required. All other plans, to my knowledge, are impossible to do for life or are unhealthy or expensive. The facts above will always hold true. And you will feel good, look good and make good progress and as a progress therapist I advocate progress or change until you do. Life is too short to stand still or regress. I once heard regression described as a living death and progression described as choosing life. Choose life – Choose progress.

Please follow our blog – www.brawnysmartypants.com

Thank you

Gary Walsh – Progress therapist – www.Soul2Whole.com (coming soon)

CONTINUE FOR OTHER WORK BY THE SAME AUTHOR

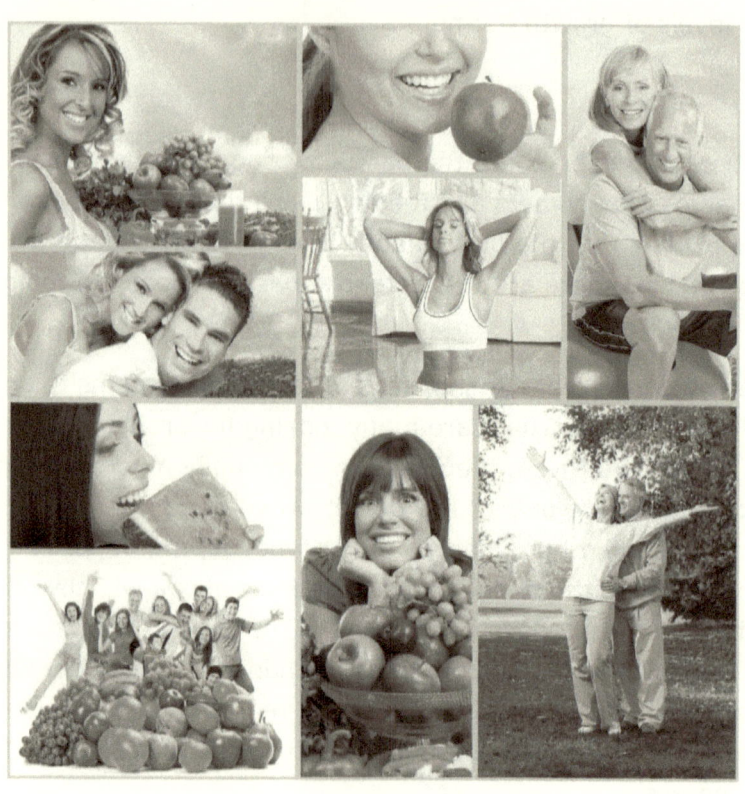

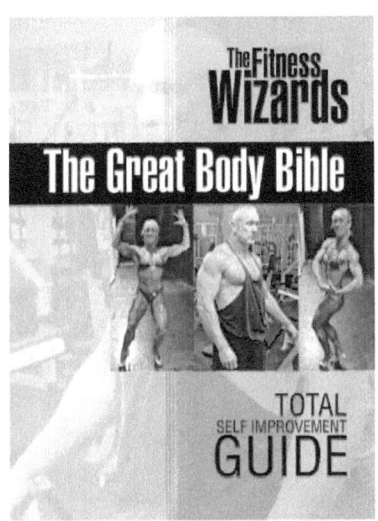

Out Now –

Walsh and Walsh, also known as the "Fitness Wizards," explore weight lifting and healthy attitudes in their debut exercise book. Despite the name, the Fitness Wizards are quite down-to-earth: "Much has been written about diet and fitness," they write, "and as often happens with a popular subject, information has become confused and often misleading." Gary Walsh, who narrates the book, and Julie, his wife, co-author and lifting partner, are upfront about the current fitness landscape: Modern life, they say, is fraught with bad food, sedentary activity, depression, body dissatisfaction and unrealistic standards of beauty. These problems are so universal that there's been no shortage of fitness prophets and self-help shamans willing to take customers' money in exchange for quick solutions. The Walshes make it clear from the start that there's no magic cure for any health issue. Health is hard, they say, and it requires a person to make serious, long-term changes in his or her life.

The authors offer a comprehensive breakdown of all aspects of physical and mental well-being, from the origins of motivation and self-discipline to an analysis of food groups and stretching strategies. The final section is a collection of memoirist and philosophical personal essays about Gary's life, career, struggles and epiphanies. There's a great deal of information on general health and an in-depth discussion of purpose and lifestyle that's applicable to any pursuit. Gary's honest, yet optimistic, voice and friendly, self-deprecating delivery are the work's strongest traits. The prose is clear and inviting. Gary is quick to remind readers that there's no one system that a person must follow to achieve his or her goals, in fitness or in life. Sometimes the thing we need the most to move forward is a sympathetic voice in our ear, and if a personal trainer is too pricey, this book might be the next best thing.

An encouraging read for anyone attempting to think healthy.

-Kirkus Indie review

Coming Soon

Soul2Whole

Countless Possibilities for Living and Personal Progress

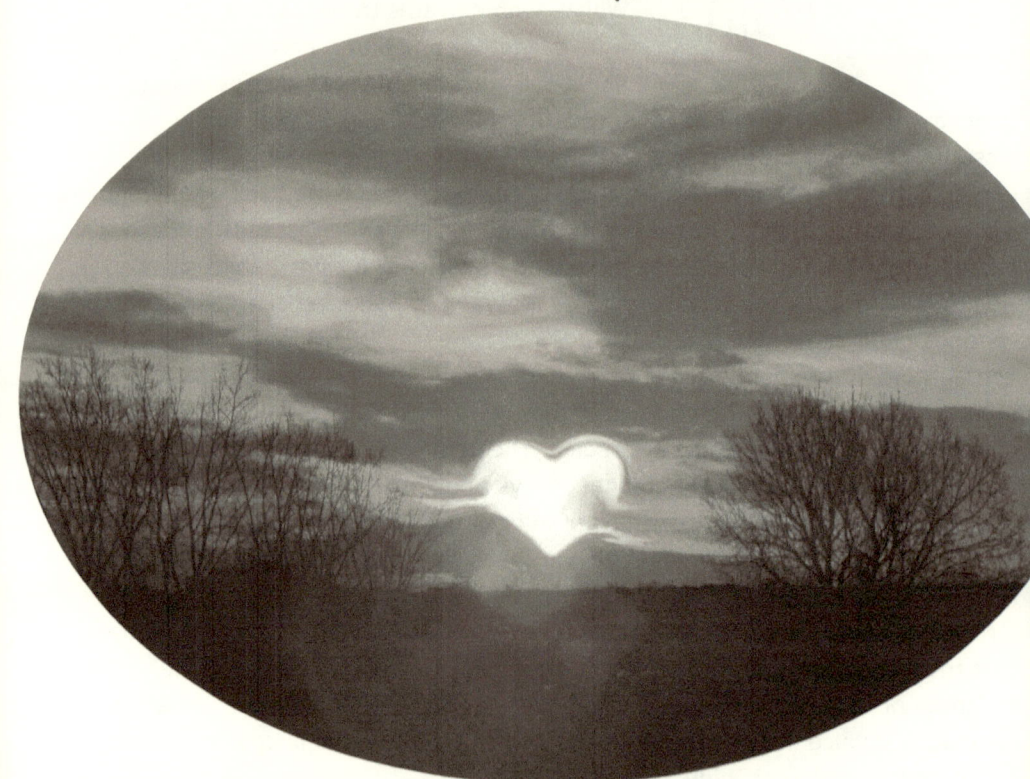

By Gary Walsh

An Introduction to Progress Therapy

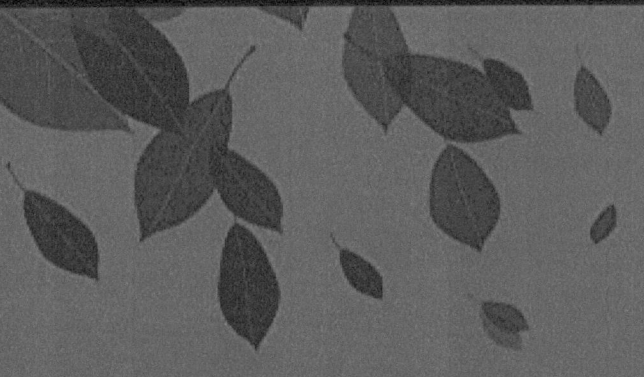

Getting Better 1
Moving In The Right Direction

Ego Busting and Enlightenment in the Real World

Gary Walsh

Out Now.

Coming Soon

SPIRIT OF PROGRESS

Signposts for Living and Personal Growth

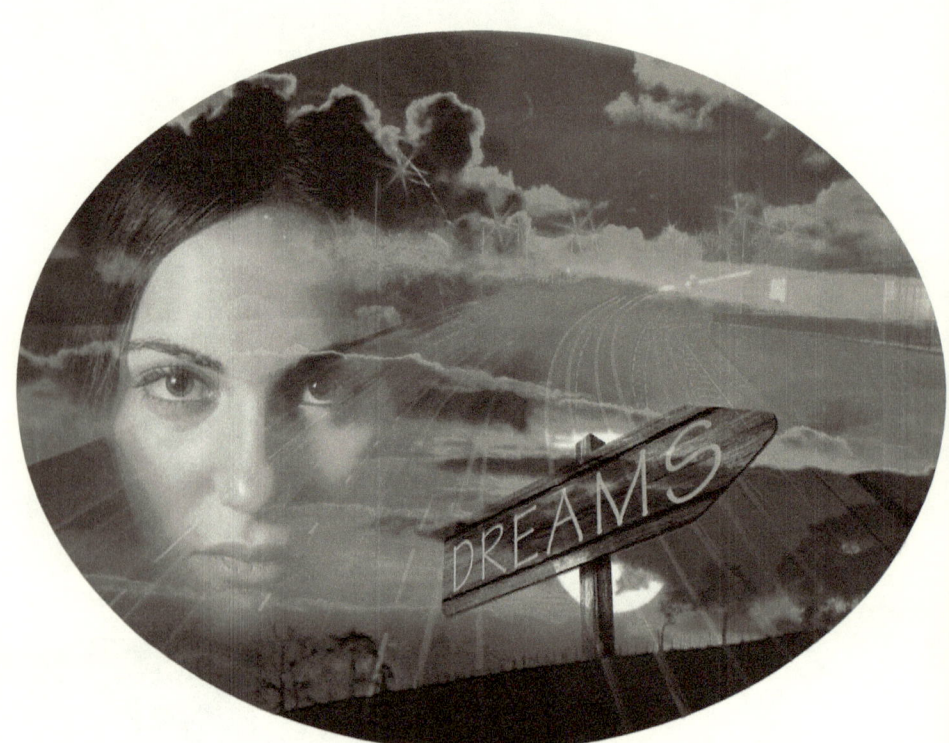

Original Thoughts
Presented By

Gary Walsh

www.ingramcontent.com/pod-product-compliance
Lightning Source LLC
Chambersburg PA
CBHW020404290526
45785CB00005B/2436